BLOOD TRANSFUSION THERAPY

A Physician's Handbook
3rd Edition

American Association of Blood Banks
1989

Editor

Patricia T. Pisciotto, MD

Contributing Editors

David Ciavarella, MD
Sanford R. Kurtz, MD
Thomas A. Lane, MD
Gary Moroff, PhD
Francis S. Morrison, MD
Stanley C. Roberts, SBB(ASCP)

Contents

Preface

The Component Therapy Committee has undertaken yet another revision of the *Physician's Handbook* in order to help keep medical and paramedical professionals aware of the ongoing changes in the field of Transfusion Medicine. The third edition is in compliance with the 13th edition of the *Standards* and virtually all sections have been updated. It includes an expanded section of leukocyte-poor components, plasma derivatives and hemostatic disorders as well as new sections on transfusion practices in transplantation and management of alloimmunization. The intent of the *Handbook* is to serve as a convenient reference for issues relating to Transfusion Medicine and, therefore, the format has remained as concise chapters with references provided for further information. As in the past, the Committee welcomes comments from the readers and also gratefully acknowledges those who have been supportive of our efforts to provide ongoing knowledge in the area of Transfusion Medicine.

Patricia T. Pisciotto, MD
Editor

SECTION I

BLOOD COMPONENTS

Concept of Blood Component Therapy

Blood component therapy refers to the transfusion of the specific part of blood that the patient needs, as opposed to the routine transfusion of whole blood. This not only conserves blood resources, since one donated unit can benefit several patients, but also provides the optimal method of transfusing patients who require large amounts of a specific blood component.

During manufacture the entire blood bag and any integrally attached satellite bags and needles are sterilized. As the entire blood collection system is sterile, disposable and never reused, it is IMPOSSIBLE for a donor to contract hepatitis, AIDS or other transfusion-transmitted diseases by donating blood. The blood collection set is considered to be a closed system, being open only at the tip of the needle used for donor phlebotomy. Once the administration ports of a blood bag are opened, however, the unit is considered to be an open system. According to the *Standards for Blood Banks and Transfusion Services*,[1] any blood component prepared in an open system and stored at 4 C has a maximum shelf life of 24 hours because of the risk of bacterial contamination. To prepare components (see Table 1) that have the maximum permitted shelf life, integral satellite bags must be used to ensure maintenance of the closed system. Alternatively, sterile connecting devices are available; these devices permit sterile attachment of separate plastic bags.

Table 1. Blood Components and Plasma Derivatives

Component/Product	Composition	Approx. Volume	Indications
Whole Blood	RBC; plasma; WBC; platelets	500 mL	increase both red cell mass and plasma volume (WBC and platelets not functional; plasma deficient in labile clotting Factors V, VIII)
Red Blood Cells	RBC; reduced plasma, WBC and platelets	250 mL	increase red cell mass in symptomatic anemia (WBC and platelets not functional)
Red Blood Cells, Adenine-Saline Added	RBC; reduced plasma, WBC and platelets; 100 mL of additive solution	330 mL	increase red cell mass in symptomatic anemia (WBC and platelets not functional)
Leukocyte-Poor RBC (prepared by filtration or centrifugation)	RBC; $<5 \times 10^8$ WBC; few platelets; minimal plasma	200 mL	increase red cell mass; prevent febrile reactions due to leukocyte antibodies; decrease the likelihood of alloimmunization to leukocyte or HLA antigens
Saline Washed RBC	RBC; $<5 \times 10^8$ WBC; no plasma	180 mL	increase red cell mass; reduce risk of allergic reactions to plasma proteins
Frozen-Thawed-Deglycerolized RBC	RBC; $<5 \times 10^8$ WBC; no platelets; no plasma	180 mL	increase red cell mass; minimize febrile or allergic transfusion reactions; used for prolonged RBC blood storage
Granulocyte-Platelet Concentrate	granulocytes; lymphocytes; platelets ($>1.0 \times 10^{10}$ PMN/unit; $>2.0 \times 10^{11}$ platelets/unit); some RBC	220 mL	provide granulocytes for selected patients
Platelet Concentrate (random donor)	platelets ($>5.5 \times 10^{10}$ platelets/unit); RBC; WBC;	50 mL	bleeding due to thrombocytopenia or thrombocytopathy

Product	Components	Volume	Indications
Platelet Apheresis	platelets ($>3 \times 10^{11}$/unit); RBC; plasma; WBC	300 mL	same as platelet concentrate; sometimes HLA matched
Fresh Frozen Plasma	plasma; all coagulation factors; complement, (no platelets)	220 mL	treatment of some coagulation disorders
Cryoprecipitate	fibrinogen; Factors VIII and XIII, von Willebrand factor	15 mL	deficiency of Factor VIII (hemophilia A) Factor XIII, fibrinogen; treatment of von Willebrand's disease
Lyophilized VIII	Factor VIII; trace amount of other plasma proteins	25 mL	hemophilia A (VIII deficiency)
Lyophilized II, VII, IX, X	Factors II, VII, IX, X	25 mL	hereditary II, VII, IX or X deficiency
Lyophilized IX	Factor IX; trace amount of other plasma proteins	25 mL	hemophilia B (IX deficiency)
Anti-inhibitor Coagulation Complex	Factor VIII bypassing activity	30 mL	patients with antibody to Factor VIII (note: indications for use not well-established)
Albumin/Plasma Protein Fraction	albumin, some α, β globulins	(5%); (25%)	volume expansion
Immune Serum Globulin	IgG antibodies	varies	treatment of hypo- or agammaglobulinemia; disease prophylaxis; autoimmune thrombocytopenia
Rh Immune Globulin	IgG anti-D	1 mL	prevention of hemolytic disease of the newborn due to D antigen
Antithrombin III	antithrombin III; trace amounts of other plasma proteins	10 mL	treatment of antithrombin III deficiency
Alpha$_1$-Proteinase Inhibitor (PI)	alpha$_1$-PI (alpha$_1$-antitrypsin); other plasma proteins	varies	congenital deficiency of alpha$_1$-PI with evidence of panacinar emphycema

Whole Blood

Description of Component

A unit of whole blood contains approximately 450 mL of blood and 63 mL of anticoagulant preservative. The hematocrit of a typical unit of blood ranges from 0.36-0.44 (36-44%). Whole blood is stored in a monitored refrigerator at 1-6 C. The shelf life of whole blood is dictated by the percent recovery of the transfused red cells 24 hours after infusion. This value must average >70%. Thus, the shelf life of whole blood depends on the preservative used in the blood collection bag [the shelf life of CPD (citrate-phosphate-dextrose) blood is 21 days; 35 days for CPDA-1 (citrate-phosphate-dextrose-adenine)]. See Table 2. 2,3-DPG 2,3-diphosphoglycerate, a molecule that facilitates the release of oxygen from hemoglobin, decreases during storage and is regenerated after infusion of the blood.[2]

There is little scientific justification for use of ''fresh'' whole blood (eg, blood collected within the previous 24 hours). Blood less than 24 hours old is rarely available, due to the time required to perform postdonation ABO and Rh typing, to screen for presence of atypical antibodies and to complete required infectious disease testing. Whole blood less than 7 days old may be desirable for neonatal exchange transfusions.

Another component, whole blood, modified, is prepared by returning the plasma to the red blood cells after removal of platelets and/or cryoprecipitate.

Indications

Whole blood provides both oxygen-carrying capacity and blood volume expansion. The primary indication is for treating patients who are actively bleeding and who have sustained a loss of greater than 25% of their total blood volume. Such a patient may develop hemorrhagic shock. Unless a patient who receives whole blood needs volume replacement in addition to oxygen-carrying capacity, fluid overload may occur, especially if rapid infusion is attempted.

Whole blood stored over 24 hours contains few viable platelets or granulocytes. In addition, levels of Factor V and Factor VIII decrease with storage. To supply platelets or granulo-

Table 2. Characteristics of Whole Blood Stored for 35 Days in CPDA-1 (N = 10)*

	Storage Time (Days)				
	0	7	14	21	35
Plasma dextrose (mg/dL)	432	374	357	324	282
Plasma sodium (mEq/L)	169	162	159	157	153
Plasma potassium (mEq/L)	3.3	12.3	17.6	21.7	17.2
Plasma chloride (mEq/L)	84	81	79	77	79
Plasma bicarbonate (mEq/L)	12.0	17.0	12.5	12.2	8.0
Whole-blood pH	7.16	6.94	6.93	6.87	6.73
Whole-blood lacate (mg/dL)	19	62	91	130	202
Plasma LDH (units)	296	1002	1222	1457	1816
Whole-blood ammonia (μg/dL)	82	280	423	521	703
Plasma hemoglobin (mg/dL)	0.5	13.1	24.7	24.7	45.6
WBC ($\chi 10^3/\mu$L)	7.2	4.0	3.0	2.8	2.4
Hematocrit (%)	35	36	35	36	36
RBC hemoglobin (g/dL)	12	12	12	12	12
RBC ($\times 10^6/\mu$L)	4.0	4.0	3.9	3.9	3.9
Red blood cell 2,3-DPG (μmol/gHb)**	13.2	—	—	—	0.7
Red blood cell ATP (μmol/gHb)**	4.18	—	—	—	2.40

* Latham JT, Bove JR, Weirich FL. Chemical and hematologic changes in stored CPDA-1 blood. Transfusion 1982;22-158-9.
** Moore, GL, Peck CC, Sohmer PR, Zuck TF. Some properties of blood stored in anticoagulant CPDA-1 solution. Transfusion 1981;21:135-7.

cytes, the appropriate cell concentrates should be used. Fresh frozen plasma should be given to replace needed labile clotting factors. Levels of stable clotting factors, however, are well-maintained in units of whole blood during storage. Whole blood, modified, has hemostatic properties similar to those of stored whole blood.

Contraindications and Precautions

Whole blood should not be given to patients with chronic anemia who are normovolemic and require only an increase in red cell mass; red blood cells should be used for such patients. Hemolytic transfusion reactions are always a risk with blood transfusion. Transmission of viral infections, such as hepatitis viruses, human immunodeficiency virus (HIV) and cytomegalovirus (CMV), as well as allergic and febrile transfusion reactions are complications that should be considered whenever blood is transfused.[3]

Dose and Administration

In an adult, one unit of whole blood will increase the hemoglobin by about 10 g/L (1 g/dL) or the hematocrit by about 0.03-0.04 (3-4%). In pediatric patients a whole blood transfusion of 8 mL/kg will result in an increase in hemoglobin of approximately 10 g/L (1 g/dL). Whole blood must be administered through a blood filter. The rate of infusion depends on the clinical condition of the patient, but each unit or aliquot should be infused within 4 hours (see p. 65).

Red Blood Cells

Description of Component

Red blood cells are prepared from whole blood by removing 200-250 mL of plasma and are stored at 1-6 C in a variety of different anticoagulant/preservative solutions. These solutions have varying amounts and/or types of preservative agents (eg, buffer, dextrose, adenine and mannitol). The resultant red blood cell components have different hematocrits and shelf lives. Red blood cells stored in additive solutions have hematocrits of 0.52-0.60 (52-60%) and a shelf life of 42 days, while red cells stored in CPDA-1 have hematocrits of 0.70-0.80 (70-80%) and can be stored for 35 days.[2,4,5] Storage of red blood cells in CPD or CP2D results in hematocrits similar to CPDA-1, but a shelf life of 21 days. Stored red blood cells do not contain functional platelets or granulocytes. Red blood cells and whole blood have the same oxygen-carrying capacity because they both contain the same number of red cells.

Indications

Red blood cells are indicated for treatment of anemia in normovolemic patients who require only an increase in oxygen-carrying capacity and red blood cell mass. These include patients with chronic anemia due to diseases such as renal failure or malignancy. The transfusion requirements of each patient should be based on clinical status rather than on any predetermined hematocrit or hemoglobin value. A volume of 500 mL of red blood cells (2 units) provides twice the increment in hematocrit, as does infusion of an equal volume of whole blood. Whole blood contains 200-250 mL of plasma, which provides an unnecessary volume load to patients who do not require or cannot tolerate excessive volume expansion, such as anemic patients with cardiac failure (especially the very young and the elderly).

Contraindications and Precautions

Risks associated with red blood cell infusion are the same as those encountered with whole blood.[3] Hypervolemia can also occur with infusion of excessive amounts of red blood cells.

Dose and Administration

Red blood cells must be transfused through a filter. The higher hematocrit of red blood cells not stored in additive solutions results in increased viscosity, which may slow the transfusion rate. Fifty to 100 mL of isotonic sodium chloride (0.9% USP) may be used to dilute the red blood cells to decrease viscosity, but this must be balanced against the risk of hypervolemia. The lower hematocrit of the additive solution red blood cell units permits more rapid infusion rates. For patients at risk of circulatory overload or for pediatric patients, concern over the additional volume due to the 100 mL of additive solution may warrant concentrating the component by centrifugation or sedimentation. No solutions other than isotonic saline, and no medications should be added to red blood cells (see p. 65).

Saline Washed Red Blood Cells

Description of Component

Red blood cells (RBCs) may be washed with sterile saline using machines specially designed for this purpose. The washed RBCs are suspended in sterile saline, usually at hematocrits of 0.70-0.80 (70-80%). Saline washing removes all but traces of plasma, reduces the concentration of leukocytes to $<5 \times 10^8$, and removes platelets and cellular debris. It may be performed at any time during the shelf life of a unit of blood, but since washing is ordinarily performed in an "open" system, the resultant packed RBCs can be stored for only 24 hours at 1-6 C.

Indications

Saline washed red cells are indicated for transfusion of patients who have had recurrent or severe allergic reactions when they are transfused with RBCs or whole blood. They may also be used in neonatal/intrauterine transfusion. Until the recent development of efficient leukocyte depletion filters (see p. 5), washed cells were frequently ordered to provide leukocyte-poor RBCs[6]; however, using washed cells for this purpose alone is, in general, no longer either necessary or justifiable.

Contraindications and Precautions

The use of an open system washing technique limits the shelf life of washed RBCs to 24 hours following preparation because of the risk of bacterial contamination.[1] Otherwise, the transfusion hazards associated with washed cells are similar to those of packed RBCs. Washed RBCs are capable of transmitting hepatitis[7] and other infectious diseases. As they contain viable lymphocytes, washed RBCs can also induce graft-vs-host disease (GVHD).

Dose and Administration

All units must be given through a blood filter. Use of saline washed red blood cells provides a smaller red cell mass to the patient due to the loss of some red blood cells during the washing procedure. Thus, patients who are chronically transfused with washed red blood cells may require additional transfusions to achieve an appropriate hematocrit.

Frozen-Thawed-Deglycerolized Red Blood Cells

Description of Component

Frozen red blood cells are prepared by adding glycerol, a cryoprotective agent, to blood usually less than 6 days old. The unit is then frozen at -65 or -200 C (depending on the concentration of cryoprotective agent) for up to 10 years. Once thawed, it is washed to remove the glycerol using a series of saline-glucose solutions. The unit is reconstituted in sterile saline, usually at hematocrits of 0.70-0.80 (70-80%), and may be stored at 1-6 C for up to 24 hours, since the washing ordinarily takes place in an "open" system.[1]

Indications

Requests for deglycerolized red blood cells have decreased over the past several years.[8] This technique is useful for storing rare units of red blood cells and for long-term preservation of red blood cells for autologous transfusion. It is not usually necessary to use deglycerolized red blood cells for routine prevention of febrile transfusion reactions nor are they useful in inventory control due to the expense and time required to store and deglycerolize such units. Their use for potential renal transplant patients has greatly declined because of information showing increased cadaver kidney graft survival in patients who are exposed to "buffy coat."[9] Frozen-thawed RBCs may be used as an alternate to CMV-negative donors in order to decrease the incidence of CMV seroconversion in susceptible patients.[10]

Contraindications and Precautions

The same risks and hazards exist as for saline washed RBCs. Frozen-thawed RBCs are capable of transmitting infectious diseases and have been shown to contain viable lymphocytes.[7]

Dose and Administration

All units must be given through a blood filter. Frozen-thawed-deglycerolized red blood cells provide a smaller red cell mass due to loss of red blood cells during processing. Therefore, patients transfused with deglycerolized red blood cells may require additional transfusions to achieve a desired hematocrit.

Platelets

PLATELET CONCENTRATES

Description of Component

Platelet concentrates are prepared from individual units of whole blood by centrifugation. Each bag should contain at least 5.5×10^{10} platelets in 50-70 mL plasma. Platelet concentrates, which are stored in the blood bank for up to 5 days at 20-24 C with constant, gentle agitation, have nearly normal posttransfusion recovery and survival.[11,12] Alternatively, they may be stored for 48 hours at 1-6 C. They are frequently pooled prior to use.

Indications

As recently reviewed at a National Institute of Health (NIH) Consensus Conference[13] platelets are indicated for treatment of bleeding due to thrombocytopenia (usually below 50×10^9/L) or to the presence of functionally abnormal platelets (thrombocytopathy). Prophylactic transfusion of platelet concentrates may be indicated for patients with platelet counts below 15-20 $\times$ 10^9/L associated with bone marrow hypoplasia due to chemotherapy, tumor invasion or primary aplasia. This number may be safely lowered for some patients.[13] There is no evidence that prophylactic transfusion of platelets is beneficial in massive transfusion[14] or in cardiac surgery.[15]

Contraindications and Precautions

Platelet transfusions are usually not effective in patients with rapid platelet destruction. These conditions include idiopathic autoimmune thrombocytopenic purpura (ITP) and untreated disseminated intravascular coagulation (DIC). In such patients platelet transfusion should be employed only in the presence of active bleeding. Patients with thrombocytopenia due to septicemia or hypersplenism may also fail to benefit from platelet transfusions.

Chills, fever and allergic reactions may occur. Fever should not be treated with antipyretics containing aspirin, as aspirin will inhibit platelet function. Repeated transfusions may lead to alloimmunization to HLA and other antigens and result in the development of a ''refractory'' state manifested by unresponsiveness to platelet transfusion (see section on Alloimmunization). Due to small amounts of red blood cells in the concentrate, Rh-negative patients should generally receive only Rh-negative platelet concentrates. If Rh-positive concentrates must be transfused to Rh-negative women of child-bearing potential, prevention of Rh immunization by the use of Rh immune globulin should be considered. Due to the plasma contained in the concentrate, ABO-incompatible platelets may cause a positive direct antiglobulin test (DAT) and, very rarely, hemolysis.[16] Such an occurrence is more likely in children due to their smaller blood volume. Rapid infusion may cause circulatory overload and other complications related to increased intravascular volume. Transfusion-transmitted diseases, of course, are an ever-present danger. Bacterial contamination of platelets is of special concern because platelets are stored at room temperature.

Dose and Administration

The usual dose for a thrombocytopenic bleeding adult is 6-10 units of concentrate; for pediatric patients it is about 1 unit/10 kg body weight. One unit of platelet concentrate usually increases the platelet count in a 70-kg adult by $5 \times 10^9/L$. Failure to achieve hemostasis or the expected increment in platelet count may signify the refractory state.[13,17] In addition to the clinical response to platelet transfusion, the emergence of antibody-mediated platelet destruction is readily ascertained by calculating the posttransfusion platelet count increment (CI):

$$CI = \frac{(\text{Post-tx plt ct}) - (\text{Pre-tx plt ct})}{\text{Platelets transfused} \times 10^{11}} \times BSA$$

where   Pre-tx plt ct = pretransfusion platelet count
            Post-tx plt ct = posttransfusion platelet count
            BSA = body surface area in square meters

A CI of $>7.5\text{-}10 \times 10^9/L$ from a sample drawn 10 minutes to 1 hour posttransfusion, or a CI of $>4.5 \times 10^9/L$ from a sample drawn 18-24 hours posttransfusion are considered acceptable, ie, not indicative of alloimmunization.[18,19] Ideally, posttransfusion counts are obtained both within 1 hour and after 18 hours; however, the early CI is more informative regarding the presence of platelet antibodies and the refractory state. The 1-hour CI is diminished primarily by antiplatelet antibodies and by splenomegaly, but the 18-24 hour CI is also diminished by fever, infection, sepsis, DIC, storage time and other factors.[20,21] Patients who repeatedly have poor clinical or 1-hour CI responses are likely to be alloimmunized, and are said to be refractory to platelet transfusion. Such patients usually require HLA-matched platelets (see section on Alloimmunization).

Platelet concentrates must be administered through a filter and pretransfusion red blood cell compatibility testing is not necessary. Concentrates may be pooled before administration or infused individually. Platelets should be transfused within 6 hours after they are pooled. Irradiation of platelets may be indicated to prevent graft-vs-host disease in immuno-suppressed or immunodeficient patients.

APHERESIS PLATELETS

Description of Component

Apheresis platelets, which are collected from an individual donor during a 2-3 hour apheresis procedure, contain more than 3×10^{11} platelets.[1] This is equal to 6-8 units of platelet concentrate. The volume of plasma in the product varies from 200-400 mL. The number of lymphocytes and red blood cells varies with the apheresis technique.

Indications

Apheresis platelets that have been HLA-matched with the recipient are indicated for patients who are unresponsive to random-donor platelet concentrates due to HLA alloimmunization. Non-HLA-matched apheresis platelets are also used in patients who are not refractory in order to limit exposure to multiple donors. Controversy exists as to whether the use of this component rather than platelet concentrate reduces the frequency of alloimmunization in patients requiring long-term platelet transfusion. In addition, there is no scientific evidence to suggest an advantage in using non-HLA-matched apheresis platelets in patients who are already alloimmunized and/or refractory unless the platelets are crossmatch-compatible.

Neither is it advantageous to use HLA-matched apheresis platelets in patients whose refractory state is not due to alloimmunization.[22] In such patients, HLA-matched apheresis platelets would not survive longer in vivo than would the random-donor platelet concentrates. Physicians treating patients refractory to platelet concentrate should consult with the transfusion service director to determine the best therapeutic alternatives (see section on Alloimmunization).

Contraindications and Precautions

Side effects and hazards are similar to those for platelet concentrates.

Dose and Administration

One unit of apheresis platelets will usually increase the platelet count of a 70-kg adult by 30-60 $\times$ 10^9/L. See above for discussion of CI. Red blood cell compatibility testing must be performed if the component contains a significant number of red blood cells ($>$5 mL). Preferably, the donor plasma should be ABO compatible with the recipient's red blood cells if they are not group-specific. Administration is similar to that for platelet concentrates.

Leukocyte-Poor Red Blood Cells and Platelets

LEUKOCYTE-POOR RED BLOOD CELLS

Description of Component

Units of whole blood or red blood cells also contain $1\text{-}3 \times 10^9$ leukocytes[6,23-27] and variable numbers of platelets. Current AABB *Standards* specifies that the method used must reduce the leukocyte contamination to $<5 \times 10^8$/unit while retaining $>80\%$ of the original red cells.[1] The standard 170-micron blood filter does not remove leukocytes. In the blood bank, leukocytes and platelets can be removed from stored blood by several methods, including inverted centrifugation followed by chilling and microaggregate filtration, by automated saline washing of liquid or previously frozen blood or by the use of special filters.[6,23]

Recently, leukocyte depletion at the bedside during blood transfusion has become possible through the use of a new generation of specially designed filters that remove $>99\%$ of leukocytes.[24,25] It should be noted that electronic particle counting, which was employed in most of the currently available reports of leukocyte depletion, has limited accuracy at the low concentrations of leukocytes remaining after filtration.[25-27] The development of improved leukocyte counting techniques is in progress and should ameliorate this problem. Leukocyte depletion by the above methods prevents or minimizes febrile reactions due to anti-leukocyte antibodies.[6,23,24] In addition, in multitransfused patients the prophylactic use of leukocyte-poor blood prepared by the new filters has been reported to diminish the likelihood of alloimmunization to leukocyte/platelet antigens.[25-27]

Indications

Leukocyte-poor red blood cells are indicated for patients who have repeated febrile reactions in association with the transfusion of red cells or platelets, and as prophylaxis against alloimmunization in selected patients who are destined to receive long-term hemotherapy. Patients who have received frequent transfusions and women who have had multiple pregnancies may become alloimmunized to leukocyte and sometimes platelet antigens.[28] This sensitization can manifest as febrile transfusion reactions and/or as refractoriness to platelet transfusion (see section on Platelets). Studies indicate that leukocytes are responsible for the development of alloimmunization to HLA antigens[29,30] and antibodies to leukocyte antigens are responsible for the majority of febrile transfusion reactions.[31,32] Most patients who have had only one febrile nonhemolytic transfusion reaction will not have a second.[32] Patients who have severe or recurrent febrile nonhemolytic transfusion reactions should receive leukocyte-poor blood components. Furthermore, since it is now possible to diminish the likelihood of alloimmunization by the routine prophylactic use of filtered leukocyte-poor blood components, patients who have a high likelihood of becoming alloimmunized (eg, patients with chronic transfusion requirements) may be considered candidates for prophylactic use of leukocyte-poor blood components.[24-26]

Decisions regarding what type of leukocyte depletion technique to use should be based on several factors including therapeutic goals (prevention of reactions in an alloimmunized patient vs prophylaxis against immunization), local experience with blood bank preparation techniques and the patient's response to previous leukocyte-poor units. Since leukocyte depletion of blood components is a rapidly evolving field, consultation with the transfusion service physician is recommended. The use of bedside filtration methods employing the new filters is successful in preventing febrile reactions in nearly all patients.[24] For patients who still experience febrile reactions, saline washed or frozen-deglycerolized red blood cells may be effective. Finally, a decision to use leukocyte-poor red blood cells prophylactically in an effort to prevent alloimmunization should be made before the first blood transfusion, and also implies a commitment to use leukocyte-poor platelets as well as red blood cells (see below).

Contraindications and Precautions

In general, leukocyte-poor red blood cells are subject to the same hazards as packed red blood cells.

Dose and Administration

Administration of red blood cells through the new bedside leukocyte depletion filters eliminates the need for the standard blood filter. Personnel who administer blood through leukocyte depletion filters should be thoroughly familiar with the requirements of their use (which vary from one filter to another) in order to achieve optimal leukocyte depletion, provide acceptable blood flow rates and ensure against excessive loss of red blood cells.

LEUKOCYTE-POOR PLATELETS

Description of Component

Platelet concentrate and apheresis platelets also contain leukocytes (approximately $0.5-1 \times 10^8$/unit of platelet concentrate),[25,26,32] which are not removed by the standard 170-micron blood filter. There are no current AABB standards for leukocyte-poor platelets; however two methods of leukocyte depletion—filtration and centrifugation—have been reported to diminish the likelihood of alloimmunization and development of the refractory state in clinical studies.[25,26,33] Leukocyte depletion may also improve platelet response in alloimmunized patients by reducing leukocyte antibody reactions and secondary destruction of platelets.[34] The number of leukocytes remaining in the component after leukocyte depletion varies with the type of platelet component (concentrate vs apheresis), the number of platelet units processed and the type of leukocyte depletion procedure employed. The new generation of filters generally remove >99% of leukocytes and less than 10% of the platelets in the platelet concentrate.[25,26] Leukocyte depletion of platelets by commercially available centrifugation methods, which remove 80-90% of leukocytes and 20-30% of platelets,[35,36] are less effective than the new filtration methods.

Indications

Leukocyte-poor platelets are indicated as prophylaxis against HLA alloimmunization in selected patients who are destined to receive long-term hemotherapy. Transfusion of leukocyte-containing blood components or pregnancy may result in the formation of alloantibodies to leukocyte (primarily HLA) antigens, which severely impair the recovery and posttransfusion survival of platelets (see discussion of CI in section on Platelets).[28] This condition is referred to as the refractory state. Recent clinical studies indicate that transfusion of leukocyte-poor blood components is associated with a significant reduction in the incidence of HLA alloimmunization and in the development of refractoriness to platelet transfusion.[24-27,33] Leukocyte depletion of platelet concentrates is most readily accomplished by the use of one of a variety of specially designed filtration devices. Use of centrifugation techniques have been associated with a decrease in alloimmunization rate in some, but not all studies.[33,35] The decision to use leukocyte-poor platelets in an effort to prevent alloimmunization should be made before the first blood transfusion, and also implies a commitment to use leukocyte-poor red blood cells.

Contraindications and Precautions

While the use of leukocyte-poor platelets may eliminate febrile reactions in patients who are already alloimmunized, their use will not improve on the low platelet recovery or short platelet survival associated with the use of random-donor platelet transfusion in such patients (see section on Alloimmunization). Other hazards are similar to those for platelets that have not been rendered leukocyte-depleted.

Dose and Administration

Personnel who prepare leukocyte-poor platelets or administer platelets through leukocyte depletion filters should be thoroughly familiar with the requirements of their use (which vary from one filter to another) in order to achieve optimal leukocyte depletion, and to ensure against excessive loss of platelets (since some filters designed for use with red cells will also remove platelets). Dose is similar to the component from which the leukocyte-poor platelets were prepared. Administration of platelets through the bedside leukocyte depletion filters eliminates the need for the standard 170-micron blood filter.

Granulocytes

Description of Component

Granulocyte concentrates are usually prepared by centrifugation leukapheresis of a single donor. Each unit contains $>1.0 \times 10^{10}$ granulocytes, variable amounts of lymphocytes, platelets and red blood cells, and is suspended in 200-300 mL of plasma. Hydroxyethyl starch (HES), a sedimenting agent, and corticosteroids may be administered to the donor to facilitate granulocyte collection. The presence of platelets in granulocyte concentrates is often beneficial, as many neutropenic patients are also thrombocytopenic. Granulocytes should be stored at 20-24 C and transfused as soon as possible, but must be infused within 24 hours of collection.[37] A variety of techniques have been employed to make "buffy coat" preparations from single units of fresh blood for neonatal granulocyte transfusion.[38]

Indications

A decision to use granulocyte concentrate should be made in consultation with the transfusion service physician. In such cases, all of the following should apply.

1. Neutropenia ($<0.5 \times 10^9$/L).
2. Fever for 24-48 hours, unresponsive to appropriate antibiotic therapy, or infection (including documented or presumed sepsis) unresponsive to antibiotics or other modes of therapy.
3. Bone marrow showing myeloid hypoplasia.
4. Patient with a reasonable chance for recovery of bone marrow function.

Granulocyte transfusions may be beneficial for septic neonatal patients[38] and patients with severe granulocyte dysfunction syndromes.[39] In such cases the indications for granulocyte transfusion are different from the above.

Contraindications and Precautions

Prophylactic use of granulocyte transfusion is of questionable therapeutic value.[40,41] The use of granulocyte transfusions is declining nationwide, as recent data have shown that appropriate antibiotic therapy may be more effective than granulocyte transfusion for infected neutropenic patients.[42] If recovery of bone marrow function is doubtful, granulocyte transfusions are unlikely to alter the clinical course of a neutropenic patient. Chills, fever and allergic reactions may occur. Slow infusion rates and the use of diphenhydramine and/or meperidine will lessen or prevent many of the side effects. Steroids and non-aspirin antipyretics (see p. 11) may be of value for treatment or prevention of febrile reactions. In some patients, severe febrile and pulmonary reactions to granulocyte concentrates may preclude their further use. The risk of disease transmission, including hepatitis, HIV and CMV infection, is present; immunization to HLA and red blood cell antigens may occur as well. In immunodeficient or immunosuppressed patients, graft-vs-host disease may occur with use of this component and irradiation of the product should be considered. The irradiation doses used to prevent GVHD do not impair the function of granulocytes.[43] Severe pulmonary insufficiency has been reported after granulocyte transfusion and controversy exists as to whether there is an increased risk of pulmonary insufficiency with the concurrent administration of amphotericin and granulocyte concentrates.[44]

Dose and Administration

Although most centers do not HLA-type granulocyte concentrates, red blood cell compatibility testing must be performed for each unit transfused because of the large number of red cells present. Studies suggest that alloimmunized patients are less likely to benefit from random-donor granulocyte concentrates.[41] There is no general agreement about the dose and duration of granulocyte transfusion therapy; however, reports on groups of patients indicate that at least 4 days of granulocyte transfusion therapy are required in order to demonstrate a beneficial effect.[41] A standard blood filter must be used.

Fresh Frozen Plasma

Description of Component

Plasma is composed primarily of water with about 7% protein and 2% carbohydrates and lipids. Fresh frozen plasma (FFP) is prepared from whole blood by separating and freezing the plasma within 6 hours of phlebotomy. It may be stored for up to one year at -18 C or lower. The volume of a typical unit is 200-250 mL. Under these conditions, loss of Factors V and VIII, the labile clotting factors, is minimal. FFP is used primarily to provide replacement coagulation factors (Table 3). One mL of FFP contains approximately one unit of coagulation factor activity.

Indications

As reviewed in a recent NIH Consensus Conference,[45] FFP is indicated for use in bleeding patients with multiple coagulation factor deficiencies secondary to liver disease, DIC and the dilutional coagulopathy resulting from massive blood or volume replacement. It is also indicated for patients with congenital factor deficiencies for which there is no coagulation concentrate available, such as deficiencies of Factor V or XI. It may be useful for patients with mild congenital and acquired factor deficiencies including mild hemophilia B (Factor IX deficiency), to reduce the risk of hepatitis associated with the use of most commercially available concentrates.

Contraindications and Precautions

FFP should not be used merely to provide blood volume expansion as this exposes patients unnecessarily to the risk of hepatitis and other transfusion-transmitted diseases. Albumin, plasma protein fraction or other colloid or crystalloid solutions are safer products to use for blood volume expansion. Similarly, FFP should not be used as a source of protein for nutritionally deficient patients. Because clotting factors are present in FFP in approximately normal concentrations of about 1 unit/mL, the posttransfusion increment in coagulation levels is limited, in part, by the patient's ability to tolerate the infused

Table 3. In Vivo Properties of Blood Clotting Factors

Factor	Plasma Concentration Required for Hemostasis	Half-life of Transfused Factor	Recovery in Blood (as % of Amount Transfused)	Stability in Liquid Plasma and Whole Blood (4 C Storage)
I (fibrinogen)	100 mg/dL	4-6 days	50%	Stable
II	40 U/dL (40%)	2-3 days	40-80%	Stable
V	10-15 U/dL (10-15%)	12 hours	80%	Unstable*
VII	5-10 U/dL (5-10%)	2-6 hours	70-80%	Stable
VIII	10-40 U/dL (10-40%)	8-12 hours	60-80%	Unstable**
IX	10-40%	18-24 hours	40-50%	Stable
X	10-15%	2 days	50%	Stable
XI	30%	3 days	90-100%	Stable
XII	—	—	—	Stable
XIII	1-5%	6-10 days	5-100%	Stable

*50% remains at 14 days.
**25% remains at 24 hours.
Adapted from Rizza ER. Management of patients with inherited blood coagulation defects. In: Bloom AL, Thomas DP, eds. Haemostasis and thrombosis. London: Churchill Livingstone, 1981:371.

volume of plasma without developing fluid overload. Accordingly, treatment of severe coagulopathies with FFP is often difficult and patients with severe coagulation factor deficiencies may need to receive more concentrated preparations if they are available.[46] In general, FFP has a risk of infectious disease transmission equal to that of whole blood. Allergic reactions including noncardiogenic pulmonary edema can occur with FFP infusion.[46,47]

Dose and Administration

The dosage of FFP depends on the clinical situation and underlying disease process. Posttransfusion assessment of the patient's coagulation status is important and monitoring coagulation function with a prothrombin time, a partial thromboplastin time or specific factor assays is critical. As with all blood components, FFP must be given through a filter. FFP is thawed at 30-37 C and should be transfused as soon as possible. After thawing, storage is at 1-6 C. Compatibility testing is not required but ABO-compatible FFP should be used.

Cryoprecipitate

Description of Component

Cryoprecipitate is a concentrated source of certain plasma proteins. It is prepared by thawing one unit of fresh frozen plasma at 4 C. After thawing, a white precipitate forms; this is the cryoprecipitate. The supernatant plasma is removed leaving the cold precipitated protein plus 10-15 mL of plasma in the bag. This material is then refrozen at -18 C or lower and has a shelf life of 1 year. Cryoprecipitate contains concentrated Factor VIII:C (the procoagulant activity), Factor VIII:vWF (von Willebrand factor), fibrinogen and Factor XIII. Each bag of cryoprecipitate contains approximately 80-120 units of Factor VIII:C, about 250 mg of fibrinogen and about 20-30% of the Factor XIII present in the initial unit.[48,49] Approximately 40-70% of the von Willebrand factor present in the initial unit of FFP is recovered in the cryoprecipitate.

Fibrinogen concentrates are no longer available due to the extremely high incidence of hepatitis associated with fibrinogen prepared from pools of human plasma. Currently, the main source of concentrated fibrinogen is cryoprecipitate.

Indications

Cryoprecipitate may be indicated for the treatment of hemophilia A, von Willebrand's disease, congenital or acquired fibrinogen deficiency, Factor XIII deficiency and obstetrical complications or other situations associated with consumption of fibrinogen, eg, DIC. It has also been reported to be beneficial in treating the bleeding tendency associated with uremia[50]; however, the use of desmopressin should be considered as initial therapy since it is free of the potential infectious complications of cryoprecipitate.[51] Small amounts of cryoprecipitate (sometimes autologous) are also used to prepare ''fibrin glue'' to aid in surgical hemostasis[52] or to remove fragmented renal calculi.[53]

Contraindications and Precautions

Cryoprecipitate should not be used to treat patients with deficiencies of factors other than Factor VIII, fibrinogen, von

Willebrand factor or Factor XIII. ABO-compatible cryoprecipitate should be used whenever possible as small amounts of anti-A and anti-B alloagglutinins are present. In rare instances, infusion of large amounts of ABO-incompatible units of cryoprecipitate can cause hemolysis; a positive DAT test can be seen with infusion of smaller doses. The risk of infectious disease transmission, for each unit of cryoprecipitate, is the same as that of FFP. When large amounts of cryoprecipitate are used the patient's fibrinogen level may become markedly elevated and should be monitored, as hyperfibrinogenemia can be associated with an increased risk of thromboembolism.

Dose and Administration

Prior to infusion, cryoprecipitate is thawed at 30-37 C. If pooled, the inside of the bags should be rinsed with a small amount of saline to maximize recovery of Factor VIII. Concentrates are administered through a standard blood filter; no compatibility test is required. If the thawed cryoprecipitate is not used immediately, it may be stored for no more than 6 hours at 1-6 C. For calculation of the dose of cryoprecipitate, see p. 72.

SECTION II

PLASMA DERIVATIVES

Factor VIII Concentrate

Description of Products

Factor VIII (referred to also as antihemophilic factor or factor VIII:C) concentrate is prepared by fractionation of pooled human plasma frozen soon after phlebotomy. There are several types of Factor VIII concentrate available. All products take the form of a sterile, stable and lyophilized concentrate. They differ in terms of protein purity and the method of treatment employed to inactivate viruses. Factor VIII concentrate has the advantage of providing a product with known dosage and small volume.

Products available are classified as having intermediate purity or high purity. The Factor VIII in intermediate purity products is approximately 1-10% of the total protein. Intermediate purity products contain some fibrinogen and other proteins. The purest products are produced with the use of murine monoclonal antibodies to a portion of the Factor VIII complex through immuno-affinity chromatography.[54,55] The purity of these products is greater than 90 prior to the addition of albumin, which is used as a stabilizer. Factor VIII produced through recombinant DNA technology is undergoing clinical evaluation.[56]

A variety of procedures are used to treat Factor VIII products to inactivate viruses and reduce the risk of infectious disease transmission. Included are different types of heat procedures and a solvent-detergent treatment involving the detergent triton X-100 and the organic solvent tri(n-butyl)-phosphate. (Both substances used in the solvent-detergent treatment procedure are removed.) The processes involved in producing monoclonal antibody purified Factor VIII also cause reduction of viruses. It should be noted that no treatment procedure(s) completely eliminates the risk of transmission of viral infections. The viral inactivation procedures reduce the level of Factor VIII that is recovered. Recent reviews on the reduction of the risk of transmission of viral infections in plasma and plasma products provide further information.[57,58]

The recovery and half-life properties of the products now available, on infusion to hemophiliacs, are comparable to those exhibited by products available in earlier years. A half-life range of 12-18 hours has been reported.[54,55] Active bleeding and inhibitors probably reduce the half-life.

Indications

Factor VIII concentrate is indicated for the treatment of hemophilia A patients (see p. 71) with moderate to severe congenital Factor VIII deficiency and for patients with low titer Factor VIII inhibitors (levels that do not exceed 10 Bethesda units per mL). Factor VIII concentrate can be infused for prophylactic or therapeutic purposes in association with preventing and controlling hemorrhage. When used for patients having inhibitors, frequent laboratory assaying of Factor VIII levels should be performed. A porcine Factor VIII material for treatment of hemophiliacs with antibodies is available.

Contraindications and Precautions

In particular, with a high dosage of an intermediate purity concentrate, marked elevations in plasma fibrinogen levels may occur. Development of a positive DAT or even hemolysis is also possible due to the presence of anti-A or anti-B alloagglutinins. Adverse reactions include malaise, fever, hives, nausea and chills. Since the highly pure concentrates have only been recently introduced, it is not known to what degree removal of extraneous proteins will reduce the extent of these adverse reactions. Concentrates prepared using a murine monoclonal antibody contain trace quantities of mouse protein and could cause antibody (hypersensitivity) against mouse protein to be formed. There is no evidence that such a phenomenon will occur other than in rare situations. As appropriate, patients should be informed about symptoms associated with hypersensitivity. Reactions due to the presence of albumin in concentrates prepared with monoclonal antibody should be rare. Factor VIII concentrate alone should not be used for treatment of von Willebrand's disease since most concentrates lack Factor VIII:vWF needed for normal platelet function.

Dose and Administration

The quantity of Factor VIII coagulant activity (VIII:C) is stated on the bottle in terms of International Units. One International

Unit is the Factor VIII activity present in one mL of normal, pooled human plasma less than 1 hour old.

The amount of lyophilized Factor VIII to be infused is determined by calculating the number of units required to achieve the desired in vivo levels and dividing by the number of units per bottle of concentrate as listed on the label. The lyophilized materials are reconstituted aseptically with the sterile diluent provided by the manufacturer and must be filtered before administration. This can be accomplished by use of an infusion set with a standard blood filter or by reconstituting the products using the filter needle provided with the product. Hospitalized patients who require repeated dosage should be monitored to ensure adequate replacement. When Factor VIII concentrates are used for treatment of patients with Factor VIII inhibitors, effectiveness of therapy should be monitored by both assay of Factor VIII levels and by evaluation of inhibitor titers. Reconstituted Factor VIII concentrates should be used a quickly as possible. The shelf life after reconstitution depends on the type of Factor VIII concentrate product.

Factor IX Concentrate

Description of Products

There are two Factor IX concentrate products available. Both are available as sterile, stable, lyophilized preparations obtained by fractionation of pooled plasma. The product that has been available for many years, traditionally referred to as prothrombin complex and now designated Factor IX Complex, contains in addition to Factor IX, some quantities of Factors II, VII and X and other proteins. The content of Factor VII in various products is quite variable. The amount of each Factor contained in each bottle is stated on the vial. The newer Factor IX product, designated Coagulation Factor IX, contains trace amounts of Factors II, VII and X. Approximately 20-30% of this product is Factor IX, while approximately 1-5% of the prothrombin complex products is Factor IX. Factor IX concentrates are now heat-treated to decrease the risk of hepatitis, HIV and other viral diseases. No procedure completely eliminates the risk of transmission of viral diseases. The half-life for Factor IX in plasma-derived products in Factor IX deficient patients has been reported to range from 24-32 hours.[59]

Indications

Factor IX concentrate products are used for treatment of patients with Factor IX deficiency known as hemophilia B, or Christmas disease (see p. 72). The prothrombin complex (Factor IX Complex) may also be of value for patients with congenital Factor VII or X deficiency. Some physicians recommend using the prothrombin complex product for treatment of patients with Factor VIII or Factor IX inhibitors.[60] When used for this indication, consultation with a physician experienced with its use is advised.

Contraindications and Precautions

Prothrombin complex products should not be used for patients with liver disease. There have been reports of thrombosis and DIC associated with use of the prothrombin complex Factor IX concentrates in patients with liver disease who can be presumed to have a deficiency of antithrombin III, and in patients with hemophilia B and hemophilia A with inhibitors to Factor VIII. The newly developed coagulation Factor IX products appear to be substantially less thrombogenic than prothrombin complex preparations. Reported side effects for prothrombin complex products include chills, fever, headache, nausea and flushing.

Dose and Administration

The quantity of Factor IX is stated on the bottle in terms of activity units. One unit is the Factor IX activity present in one mL of normal human plasma. The dosage needed depends on the characteristics and symptoms of the patient. The amount of concentrate to be infused to raise Factor IX levels is determined by calculating the number of units required to achieve the desired in vivo levels. Factor IX concentrate needs to be aseptically reconstituted with a sterile diluent provided by the manufacturer. Reconstituted material must be filtered before use. It needs to be infused intravenously as soon as possible after reconstitution within the time limit established for a particular product. The in vivo recovery is approximately 50%.

Anti-Inhibitor Coagulation Complex (AICC)

Description of Product

AICC is prepared by fractionation of pooled human plasma. It is a stable, sterile product containing what has been termed Factor VIII inhibitor bypassing activity. Although the exact substance(s) responsible for its clinical effect has (have) not been identified, it consists of activator and precursor vitamin K coagulation factors including activated Factor VII and Factor X. AICC is heat-treated to reduce the risk of transmission of hepatitis, HIV and other viral diseases.

Indications

AICC is indicated for patients with a high titer Factor VIII inhibitor.[60,61] Overall, 10-15% of individuals with hemophilia A and 1-2% of individuals with hemophilia B develop inhibitors. Patients with a Factor VIII inhibitor titer over 10 Bethesda units are considered candidates for treatment. This product should be used cautiously and a physician experienced in its use should be consulted prior to infusion. The effectiveness of this material has varied.[60] Both hemophilic and nonhemophilic patients exhibiting inhibitors to the Factor VIII molecule have been treated. It has also been used to treat serious bleeding episodes in patients with Factor IX inhibitors.[60]

Contraindications and Precautions

The risk of thrombosis and DIC are high and the patient should be monitored for these complications. Signs of hypotension may also occur with AICC. Special caution should be exercised when using this product with newborns and individuals with liver disease. Adverse reactions are similar to those discussed under Factor VIII. As with other products such as Factor VIII or Factor IX concentrates, the treatment to inactivate viruses does not completely eliminate the risk of transmission of viral infections.

Dose and Administration

The activity of this product is included on the bottle label. One unit refers to the amount of activated prothrombin complex which, on addition, to Factor VIII inhibitor or deficient plasma, will correct the partial thromboplastin clotting time to 35 seconds. The dosage to be used depends on the severity of the condition. AICC needs to be aseptically reconstituted with a sterile diluent provided by the manufacturer. Reconstituted material must be filtered before use. It needs to be infused as soon as possible after reconstitution within the product time limit. Adverse reactions are similar to those discussed under Factor VIII.

14

Albumin and Plasma Protein Fraction

Description of Product

Albumin is derived from donor plasma obtained either from whole blood or from plasmapheresis. It is composed of 96% albumin and 4% globulin and other proteins. Prepared by the cold alcohol fractionation process, both derivatives are subsequently heated to 60 C for 10 hours. These products do not transmit viral diseases because of the extended heating period. Plasma protein fraction (PPF) is a similar product except that it is subjected to fewer purification steps in the fractionation process. PPF contains about 83% albumin and 17% globulins. Normal serum albumin is available as a 25% or a 5% solution, while PPF is available as a 5% solution. Each has a sodium content of about 145 mmol/L (145 mEq/L). The 5% solution is osmotically and oncotically equivalent to plasma, while the 25% solution is five times that of plasma. These products can be stored for up to 5 years at 2-10 C.

Indications

In general, patients receiving albumin or PPF should be both hypovolemic and hypoproteinemic. The appropriate use of albumin is described in Table 4.[62,63] Its use in the adult respiratory distress syndrome (ARDS) is controversial. Indications for use of PPF parallel those given for 5% albumin.

Contraindications of Precautions

Use of the 25% albumin solution is contraindicated in dehydrated patients unless it is supplemented by the infusion of crystalloid solutions to provide volume expansion. Both albumin and PPF should be used with caution in patients susceptible to fluid overload. Reported side effects include flushing, urticaria, chills, fever and headache. Rapid infusion of PPF at rates over 10 mL/min has produced hypotension attributed both to sodium acetate and Hageman-Factor fragments.[64] PPF is contraindicated for intraarterial administration or infusion during cardiopulmonary bypass. Albumin does not have this restriction.

Table 4. Indications for Use of Albumin

Use	Indication for Use Appropriate?	
Plasma exchange/dialysis	YES	— to support blood pressure
Hemolytic disease of newborn	YES	— to bind indirect bilirubin during exchange transfusion
Protein losing nephropathy/enteropathy	YES	— to induce diuresis in fluid overload (use in combination with a diuretic)
	YES	— to raise blood pressure if acutely hypotensive
	NO	— to raise serum albumin
Burns	YES	— after first 24 hours if hypoproteinemia develops
	NO	— for first 24 hours
Acute/chronic liver failure	YES	— to induce diuresis in fluid overload (use in combination with a diuretic)
	YES	— to raise blood pressure if acutely hypotensive
	NO	— to raise serum albumin
Ascites	YES	— if hypotensive after paracentesis
	NO	— to mobilize ascites
Shock (nonhemorrhagic)	YES	— if total protein is <52 g/L (<5.2 g/dL)
	NO	— if total protein is >52 g/L (>5.2 g/dL) use crystalloid instead
Adult respiratory distress syndrome	YES	— if total protein is <52 g/L (<5.2 g/dL)
	NO	— crystalloid probably better
Nutritional support	NO	— use TPN or oral feeding
Wound healing	NO	— unless used to reduce peripheral edema in hypoproteinemic patient

Dose and Administration

Albumin and PPF need not be given through a filter. No compatibility testing is required since no ABO blood group antigens or antibodies are present. The dosage of albumin or PPF is determined as that amount necessary to maintain the circulating plasma protein level at 52 g/L (5.2 g/dL) or greater. Albumin will not correct chronic hypoalbuminemia, however, and should not be used for long-term therapy. The only rate restrictions apply to infusion of PPF (see above).

15

Synthetic Volume Expanders

Description of Products

Crystalloid solutions such as normal saline and Ringer's lactate are composed of various anions and cations. They are isotonic and isosmotic with plasma. Normal saline contains only sodium and chloride ions, while Ringer's lactate also contains potassium, calcium and lactate. The lactate provides buffering capacity in that it is metabolized to bicarbonate. Hypotonic solutions of sodium chloride are also available.

Colloid substitutes useful for volume expansion include Dextran and hydroxyethyl starch (HES). Dextrans are branched-chain polysaccharides composed of glucose units. They are available in low molecular weight (Dextran 40) and a high molecular weight (Dextran 70) class. HES is derived from a waxy starch composed of amylopectin. Hydroxyethyl ether groups are chemically introduced into the glucose units to retard degradation by amylase. HES is available as a 6% solution in normal saline.

Indications

By virtue of their oncotic properties, both Dextran and HES tend to stay within the vascular compartment, and thus are useful as volume expanders in hemorrhagic shock or burn shock. Crystalloid solutions will expand the plasma volume temporarily since only one-third of the salt solution remains in the intravascular space.[65] Accordingly, to replace one volume of lost plasma, two to three volumes of crystalloid are required. Crystalloid solutions are useful in patients with shock due to hemorrhage or burns where it is necessary to rapidly expand the plasma volume. In burn patients, crystalloid is the treatment of choice for volume expansion in the first 24 hours as the capillary leak in the burned areas renders albumin ineffective as an oncotic agent. Crystalloid solutions, Dextran and HES are relatively nontoxic and inexpensive, readily available, can be stored at room temperature, require no compatibility testing and are free of the risk of transfusion-transmitted disease. The controversy over the use of saline solutions (crystalloid) versus colloid for acute hypovolemia has existed for many years. A recent report provides an update on the issues of the controversy.[66]

Side Effects and Precautions

Dextran can produce anaphylactic reactions, fever, rash, tachycardia or hypotension. In addition, due to Dextran's interference with platelet function and its stimulation of fibrinolysis, its use is associated with increased bleeding tendencies. Renal failure has been reported with infusion of the low molecular weight products. The side effects due to HES occur less frequently than those reported for Dextran, but include prolongation of prothrombin and partial thromboplastin times as well as pruritus. All volume expanders require consideration of the possibility of fluid overload in patients with congestive heart failure or anuric renal failure.

Administration

Crystalloid solutions, Dextran and HES do not need to be administered through a blood filter.

16

Immune Serum Globulin

Description of Products

Immune serum globulins may be concentrated by cold ethanol fractionation from pools of human plasma. The method of fractionating immune serum globulins results in a sterile product that is also free of the risk of virus transmission (eg, hepatitis B virus and HIV). Until recently, gammaglobulin preparations and specific preparations with high titers against specific antigens were available only for intramuscular use (IMIG). These products have a number of disadvantages including the following: intramuscular administration requires 4-7 days to achieve effective plasma levels; the maximum dose that can be given is limited by muscle mass; administration may be painful; and in vivo preparations can undergo proteolytic breakdown at the intramuscular site.[67] Intramuscular products are now given primarily for disease prophylaxis. Intramuscular preparations are sterile solutions with protein concentrations of approximately 165 g/L (16.5 g/dL). The predominant immunoglobulin is IgG, but IgA and IgM may also be present.

There are now available intravenous gammaglobulin preparations (IVIG) in which the disadvantages of IMIG preparations are minimized. They are prepared as sterile lyophilized preparations or solutions which differ in mode of preparation, use of additives and pH.[67,68] Vials contain stated amounts of protein between 0.5 and 10 g. Over 90% of the protein is IgG gammaglobulin; there are only trace quantities of IgA and IgM. The IVIG products provide a way of achieving peak levels of IgG immediately after infusion. The gammaglobulin molecules of IVIG preparations are intact.

The half-lives of IV and IM preparations have been reported to vary from 18-32 days[67] or the same as native IgG.

Indications

There are a number of specific clinical uses for immune serum globulin preparations.[69] They can be used to provide passive antibody prophylaxis to susceptible individuals exposed to certain diseases and as replacement therapy for primary immunodeficiency states such as congenital agammaglobulinemias, common variable immunodeficiency, Wiskott-Aldrich syndrome and severe combined immunodeficiency.[67,70] Intravenous preparations can be used to treat selected patients (child and adult) with acute and chronic idiopathic thrombocytopenic purpura (ITP).[71,72] Recent studies indicate IV preparations can be used in treating AIDS-related thrombocytopenia[72] and for prophylactic purposes with bone marrow recipients. Other promising specific uses for the IV preparations have recently been reviewed.[67]

Contraindications and Precautions

Adverse reactions to immune serum globulin preparations can include headache, fatigue, chills, backache, lightheadedness, fever, flushing and nausea. There is the possibility of immediate hypersensitivity and anaphylactic reactions (especially if IM preparations are inadvertently given IV). Individuals with a history of IgA deficiency (with anti-IgA) or severe anaphylactic reactions to plasma products should not, in general, receive immune serum globulins. The intramuscular preparation must not be given intravenously. It has recently been concluded that gammaglobulin products ''are remarkably safe'' and that ''all preparations as now manufactured would appear to be safe from HIV and probably hepatitis B transmission.''[73,74] Non-A,non-B hepatitis has rarely been observed following use of some preparations of IVIG.[74,75]

Dose and Administration

The dose of immune globulin is dependent on the reason for administration, patient characteristics and whether an IM or IV preparation is utilized. Some of the recommended dose schedules are as follows:

Congenital immunoglobulin deficiencies
    IM—0.7 mL/kg monthly
    IV—100 mg (2 mL)/kg monthly
Prophylaxis for hepatitis A: 0.02-0.04 mL/kg IM
Hyperimmune globulins for specific diseases
    Hepatitis B—0.06 mL/kg IM: repeat at 1 month
    Varicella zoster—1 vial (2.5 mL)/10 kg (maximum of 5
    vials), IM; should be given within 72 hours of exposure
Rh immune globulin (see section on Rh immune globulin)

17

Rh Immune Globulin (RhIG)

Description

Rh immune globulin is prepared from plasma of human donors who have become immunized to Rh-positive red blood cells. The product contains predominantly IgG anti-D in a volume of about 1 mL. Each standard dose vial (300 μg) will protect against 15 mL of Rh-positive red blood cells (30 mL whole blood). The "micro-dose" vial (50 μg), which is protective for up to 5 mL of whole blood or 2.5 mL of red blood cells, is also available. The "micro-dose" vial is mainly used for first trimester bleeding, abortion or miscarriage (see below).

Indications and Dosage

Antepartum

For Rh-negative women, a "micro-dose" vial of RhIG is protective for abortion, miscarriage, vaginal hemorrhage, ectopic pregnancy or abdominal trauma occurring during the first 12 weeks of gestation. After 12 weeks of gestation a standard dose vial of RhIG should be administered for such complications. A standard dose vial is recommended for use after amniocentesis.[76] If repeated amniocentesis is performed, repeated dosages should be considered.

Most authorities recommend that all unimmunized Rh-negative women receive a standard dose of Rh immune globulin around 28 weeks of gestation. This has been shown to reduce by about 90% the approximately 1% of Rh-negative woman who become immunized during gestation.[77,78]

Postpartum

All unsensitized Rh-negative women delivering Rh-positive infants should receive one standard dose vial of Rh immune globulin unless previous maternal immunization to the D antigen has been demonstrated. Postpartum, a maternal blood sample must be drawn and evaluated for fetal-maternal hemorrhage on all Rh-negative women. In about one in 300 cases, fetal-maternal hemorrhage will exceed 15 mL of red blood cells and one or more additional doses of Rh immune globulin will be required.

Rh immune globulin should be administered to Rh-negative women even when their serum contains blood group antibodies other than anti-D. If antepartum Rh immune globulin has been administered, an additional maternal postpartum dose of 300 μg is required if the infant is Rh-positive. Antepartum administration may cause a positive antibody screen in the mother, which must not be interpreted as active immunization. Here, as in other areas of medicine, obtaining a good patient history is essential.

Administration

Rh immune globulin should be administered intramuscularly to the mother within 72 hours of delivery of the possible immunizing event. If more than 72 hours elapse, the dose should be given since it may still be protective.

Special Considerations

Rh immune globulin may also be given when Rh-positive blood products are given to Rh-negative women of childbearing potential. One standard dose vial is sufficient to protect against the red blood cells contained in more than 10 units of platelet concentrate. Administration of multiple vials of Rh immune globulin for the inadvertent or unavoidable infusion of Rh-positive red blood cells to an Rh-negative recipient has been recommended, but this is generally impractical when more than one unit of blood has been transfused, for example, during treatment of hemorrhage or major trauma. Twenty μg of RhIG per mL of red blood cells should be given within 72 hours. There have been no reports of HIV transmission with use of intramuscular globulin preparations such as Rh immune globulin.[73,79]

In a limited number of case reports, infusion of RhIG in Rh-positive patients with chronic or acute immune thrombocytopenia has resulted in a transient but significant rise in platelets. The mechanism and role of this treatment require further study.[80]

There appears to be no risk associated with administration of excessive amounts of RhIG to Rh-negative individuals. However, inadequate RhIG therapy may enhance the likelihood of alloimmunization. This is known as augmentation of primary Rh alloimmunization.[81]

Antithrombin III Concentrate

Description of Product

Antithrombin III concentrate, a recently introduced plasma derivative, is prepared by fractionation of large pools of human plasma. This lyophilized product is treated with heat to reduce the risk of transmission of viral diseases. It should be noted that no treatment procedure completely eliminates the risk of transmission of viral infections. The half-life has been determined to be approximately 60-70 hours but is shorter during heparin treatment.

Indications

Antithrombin III is an important inhibitor of coagulation. It is required for heparin to act as an anticoagulant (see p. 75). Thrombin and other Factors (IX, X, XI and XII) are inhibited by its action. Antithrombin III preparations are used to treat congenital deficiency, which is associated with thrombotic disease.[82] This product should be infused to reduce the risk of thrombosis when the blood antithrombin III level is below 75% of normal. There are a number of variant types of antithrombin deficiency. There are other potential uses for antithrombin III.

Contraindications and Precautions

The response to heparin is restored during antithrombin therapy. Heparin dose may need to be lowered during treatment to reduce the risk of bleeding. Vasodilation may occur in patients with DIC. Allergic reactions may occur.

Dose and Administration

The dosage of antithrombin III is determined to increase the circulating level to between 80% and 120% of normal. The lyophilized material must be aseptically reconstituted with the sterile solution provided by the manufacturer prior to infusion. Antithrombin III activity after therapy should be monitored using an appropriate laboratory procedure.

Alpha$_1$-Proteinase Inhibitor Concentrate

Description of Product

Alpha$_1$-proteinase inhibitor (also known as alpha$_1$-antitrypsin), a recently introduced plasma derivative, is prepared by fractionation of pooled plasma. The product is a sterile, stable and lyophilized preparation. Alpha$_1$-proteinase inhibitor is heat-treated to decrease the risk of hepatitis, HIV and other viral diseases. However, no procedure completely eliminates the risk of transmission of viral diseases. Alpha$_1$-proteinase inhibitor concentrate contains small amounts of other plasma inhibitors including alpha$_2$-plasmin inhibitor, alpha- antichymotrypsin, C$_1$-esterase and antithrombin III. The half-life of alpha$_1$-proteinase inhibitor is approximately 4.4 days.[83]

Indications

The genetic disorder associated with reduced alpha$_1$-proteinase inhibitor is referred to as alpha$_1$-antitrypsin deficiency. There are a number of different phenotypes of the deficiency. The main clinical manifestation of alpha$_1$-proteinase inhibitor deficiency is pulmonary emphysema, in which reduced levels of the protein are present in the blood and lungs. This protein acts by inhibiting neutrophil elastase, a protease that has the capability of destroying connective tissue components of the lung parenchyma. Individuals with serum levels less than 35% of normal have insufficient amounts of this protein for protecting against elastase damage.[84]

Alpha$_1$-proteinase inhibitor is used with patients having severe congenital deficiency of the protein in association with clinically demonstrable panacinar emphysema.[83,85]

Contraindications and Precautions

Administration of alpha$_1$-proteinase inhibitor appears to be well-tolerated. In clinical studies, rare adverse reactions reported included delayed fever, light-headedness, dizziness and mild transient leukocytosis. The manufacturer's instructions recommend that recipients be immunized against hepatitis B, even though the product is heat-treated.[83]

Dose and Administration

The functional activity, in milligrams, determined by inhibition of porcine pancreatic elastase, is stated on the label of each vial. Caution should be used when serum assay results are expressed in terms of antigenic activity. The recommended dosage of active protein is 60 mg/kg body weight administered intravenously once weekly.[25] Alpha$_1$-proteinase inhibitor should be reconstituted using instructions provided by the manufacturer.

20

Blood Transfusion Alternatives

Acellular Oxygen-Carrying Substances

There is no currently available artificial oxygen-carrying red blood cell substitute (commonly termed blood substitute). Substantial efforts to develop a red cell substitute are ongoing. Three types of products are being developed. One group of preparations consists of intramolecular crosslinked or poly-merized hemoglobin. A compound such as pyridoxal phosphate is incorporated into the hemoglobin molecule to allow efficient off-loading of oxygen. Products containing hemoglobin encapsulated into phospholipid liposomes and new types of perfluorocarbon emulsions are also being developed. Although there have been substantial studies with the artificial perfluorocarbon Fluosol DA emulsion,[86] including trans-fusions to individuals refusing blood transfusions on religious grounds, this product does not appear to be suitable for human use.

Recombinant Human Hematopoietic Factors

Erythropoietin is the protein-hormone that ensures the mainte-nance of satisfactory levels of red cells.[87] Its normal produc-tion is reduced in patients with kidney disease. Erythropoietin prepared by recombinant DNA technology has been shown to stimulate red cell production in anemic patients with end-stage renal disease[88-90] and is now approved for use in such patients. Recombinant human erythropoietin (r-HuEPO) therapy has been shown to be safe and well-tolerated. A phase III clinical trial found that nearly all dialysis patients exhibited target hematocrit levels (approximately 0.35 or 35%) within 8-12 weeks of the initiation of treatment. The protein was adminis-tered three times weekly following dialysis. By 12 weeks of treatment, almost no units of red cells were required. The need for red cell transfusion was eliminated in the overwhelming number of patients.[90] The major adverse effect pertains to the increase in blood pressure, which can be managed with anti-hypertensive medication.[90] Patients receiving erythropoietin also may require iron supplementation to prevent iron deficiency.

Recombinant human granulocyte colony-stimulating factor (rhG-CSF) and granulocyte macrophage colony-stimulating factor (rhGM-CSF) have been shown in clinical trials to stimulate myelopoiesis, as well as possible stimulation of certain myeloid function.[90] Further evaluation of these factors, as well as potential side effects, are still under investigation.

SECTION III

TRANSFUSION PRACTICES

Maximal Surgical Blood Order Schedule/ Type and Screen

Otherwise healthy adult patients with a normal hemoglobin level who are undergoing elective surgical procedures do not usually require blood replacement if there is less than 1000 mL of blood loss, provided that intravascular volume is maintained with crystalloid or colloid solutions. In fact, only 9% of all surgical patients actually receive blood transfusions.

A maximal surgical blood order schedule (MSBOS) can improve utilization of blood resources, increase efficiency of blood bank personnel (who use the list rather than depend on orders for each case) and decrease patient care costs by eliminating unnecessary crossmatches.[91] The schedule is developed by analyzing blood usage for each specific elective surgical procedure and comparing the number of units crossmatched to the number of units transfused, the crossmatch/transfusion (C/T) ratio. Those surgical procedures that have C/T ratios greater than 2.5 are considered to have an excessive number of units of blood ordered. The goal of the MSBOS is to limit the number of units crossmatched to the usual number transfused. MSBOS schedules will vary among different institutions.

For surgical procedures with an average usage of less than 0.5 unit of blood per operation, a type and screen procedure is recommended.[92] With a type and screen, the transfusion service determines the patient's ABO group and Rh type, and performs an antibody screen. Clinically significant antibodies, if detected, are identified and blood lacking the corresponding antigen(s) is crossmatched. On the rare occasion when blood is required for one of these low blood use procedures, patients who have a negative antibody screen can receive ABO and Rh type-specific blood, which has a 99.7% likelihood of being compatible.[93]

Development and acceptance of MSBOS and type and screen programs for elective surgery requires a close working relationship between the transfusion service, surgeons and anesthesia personnel.

Autologous Transfusion

Preoperative Autologous Donation

Autologous transfusion is the process of collection, storage and reinfusion of the patient's own blood. All patients who must undergo elective surgical procedures for which blood replacement is anticipated should be considered candidates for preoperative blood donation since it represents the safest source of transfusion. Advantages include the elimination of infectious disease transmission; risk of alloimmunization to red blood cell, platelet and leukocyte antigens; and the risk of hemolytic, febrile, allergic or graft-vs-host reactions. It can provide a source of blood for persons who have rare blood types or antibodies that make it difficult to find compatible blood. Some persons who refuse blood from homologous donors because of religious or other beliefs may accept their own blood.

Participants should be familiar with all aspects of a preoperative autologous donation program such as which blood components will be collected and stored. Patients must understand that involvement in such a program does not guarantee transfusion with only their own blood because unexpected blood loss or inability to collect the desired number of units may occur. Unlike volunteer blood donors, there are no permanent deferral (general information or history criteria) for autologous-only donation. There are no specific requirements as to age; therefore, both elderly patients and children less than 17 years of age can participate in an autologous donation program. Depending on the patient's weight, it may be necessary to reduce the volume of blood withdrawn at each donation.[94] In addition, obstetrical patients can donate after the 13th week of gestational age, with most donations occurring in the third trimester.[95]

It is the responsibility of the transfusion service physician to carefully evaluate the safety of patient donation. The hematocrit should not be less than 0.33 (33%) [hemoglobin 110 g/L (11.0 g/dL)] prior to donation. First-time autologous donors who are anemic must be evaluated by a physician to determine the cause of the anemia before the first unit can be drawn. Not all patients will be acceptable candidates for preoperative autologous donation because of concurrent medical problems. The few clinical conditions that are considered contraindications to autologous donation include severe aortic stenosis, recent myocardial infarction, unstable angina, severe hypertension and bacteremia.

Autologous units are usually stored in the liquid state at 1-6 C for 35-42 days, depending on the anticoagulant/preservative used. If more prolonged storage is needed, units can be frozen, presuming the technology is available nearby. A common schedule is to donate one unit of blood per week. In adults, the last unit is donated no closer than 72 hours before surgery to avoid hypovolemia at the time of surgery. All patients donating more than one unit of blood should receive oral iron supplementation.

Cancellation or postponement of elective surgical procedures is not uncommon, so a system must be established to ensure communication between the patient, transfusion service and the patient's physician. Under utilization of preoperative autologous blood donation for transfusion appears to be widespread. Orthopedic surgery accounts for the vast majority of these donor patients, followed by plastic surgery. These participants, however, represent only a small percentage of eligible patients having surgical procedures. Controversy exists regarding the safety of providing unused autologous blood products for allogeneic transfusion and practices differ among institutions. To ''crossover'' an autologous unit the donor must meet standard volunteer blood donation criteria. Some studies have reported an increased incidence of abnormal hepatitis serology results or less reliable medical histories from autologous donors but this has not been confirmed in other studies.[96] Before transfusion, the patient and the autologous units should have the ABO group and Rh type confirmed.

Intraoperative Salvage

Intraoperative salvage is an approach to blood conservation that involves collection and reinfusion of shed blood lost intraoperatively or from an extracorporeal circuit. Using this technique, patients can receive their own blood salvaged from the operative field and minimize the need for allogeneic blood. Various types of devices are available for retrieval of blood from the operative site. Intraoperative blood salvage is contraindicated when there is a risk of the blood being contaminated with bacteria or tumor cells. All salvaged blood must be filtered before reinfusion. Most protocols provide for washing the red blood cells before reinfusion; this removes fibrin, activated clotting factors, cellular debris, free hemoglobin, potassium and other metabolites. Blood collected by intraoperative salvage cannot be transfused into other patients, must be filtered and can be stored for no longer than 6 hours at 1-6 C before infusion.[1]

Intraoperative Hemodilution

Another form of intraoperative salvage involves hemodilution. Prior to cardiopulmonary bypass or other surgery, 1-3 units of the patient's blood can be removed and stored in approved plastic blood collection bags. The volume of blood removed is replaced with crystalloid and/or colloid solutions. As a result, blood with a lower hematocrit is lost during surgery. Perioperatively the patient's own blood is reinfused. This procedure not only helps restore the individual's red cell mass but provides viable platelets and clotting factors since the blood has been stored for only a few hours. This type of intraoperative salvage requires close patient monitoring to guard against fluid overload as well as attention to technique to ensure that the blood is collected in a sterile manner and properly labeled and stored.

Postoperative Salvage

Techniques are also available for salvaging blood collected postoperatively such as blood obtained from chest tube or joint cavity drainage. This blood is defibrinated, unclottable and contains high titers of fibrinogen-fibrin degradation products. The blood collected is processed with or without cell washing and filtered prior to reinfusion. Blood intended for retransfusion must be transfused within 6 hours of collection.

Emergency Transfusion

Description and Indications

Emergency transfusion refers to the urgent need for blood administration to ensure a patient's survival. Critical factors include the need to halt massive hemorrhage, replace intravascular volume and reestablish oxygen-carrying capacity. Most authorities recommend immediate intravascular volume repletion with crystalloid or colloid solutions.[97] If volume replacement leads to clinical stabilization, transfusion becomes less urgent and should await the completion of ABO grouping, Rh typing and compatibility testing. If the patient's vital signs and clinical condition do not rapidly stabilize, group-specific or group-compatible red blood cells should be infused as soon as available even though pretransfusion compatibility testing may not be completed.

Treatment Strategy and Risks

Delay in the provision of blood to complete standard pretransfusion testing may at times jeopardize the patient. In such circumstances blood must be issued prior to completion of routine processing or compatibility testing. The patient's physician must sign a statement indicating the nature of the emergency either before or after the blood is issued. If the patient has been previously tested by the blood transfusion service and the antibody screen is negative, the transfusion of uncrossmatched, but ABO- and Rh-compatible whole blood or red blood cells is as safe as crossmatched blood approximately 99.7% of the time.[93] This margin of safety is dependent, however, on the correct identification of the patient, the pretransfusion blood sample and the blood components to be infused. The approach to emergency transfusion in a patient who has already received blood and has had multiple specimens tested is different than that in a patient who has no previous transfusion record and has had no blood specimens analyzed.

Selection of Transfusion Products

Only ABO-group-specific whole blood should be transfused when whole blood is needed. Group O Rh-negative red blood cells should be used when the patient's blood type is unknown, particularly in women of childbearing age.

Massive Transfusion

Description

Massive transfusion is defined as the replacement of one or more blood volumes within 24 hours. A blood volume is estimated as 75 mL/kg or about 5000 mL (10 or more units of whole blood) in a 70-kg adult. There is little evidence that the numerous metabolic, coagulation, respiratory and other complications ascribed to massive transfusion are due solely to the transfusion of stored blood.[97,98] Most complications attributed to massive transfusion are actually due to tissue damage or hypoperfusion secondary to trauma or hemorrhage.

Selection of Components

Massive transfusion is an indication for the use of whole blood. However, red blood cells reconstituted with crystalloid or colloid solutions are also adequate for restoring blood volume and oxygen-carrying capacity.[99] The patient's past history, vital signs, clinical situation and hematocrit will determine the urgency with which red cell support is given. Plasma and platelet concentrate support should be based on the presence or absence of microvascular (not surgical) bleeding and on the results of screening tests of hemostasis (PT, PTT, fibrinogen and platelet count). The clinical efficacy of pre-established formulas to guide component replacement, such as giving one unit of FFP or fresh whole blood with every 5 units of red blood cells, has never been established. These formulas provide insufficient support to patients with consumptive coagulopathies (DIC) and unnecessary components to most patients, who do not develop DIC. By monitoring laboratory tests of hemostasis, the transfusion of platelets, plasma or cryoprecipitate can be reserved for patients with documented deficiencies.

Factor V and VIII levels, although diminished in stored blood, remain at hemostatic levels in the massively transfused patient unless an accelerated consumptive process is present. When transfusing whole blood, significant dilution of these factors is not seen unless 3-4 blood volumes have been replaced. Comparable data are not available when red blood cells rather than whole blood are given, and dilutional coagulopathy may occur earlier in this setting. Mild-to-moderate prolongations of the PT or PTT do not accurately predict subhemostatic clotting factor levels. Marked (>1.7 times control) prolongations of these tests are often due to factor levels below 20-30%, however, and supplemental FFP or cryoprecipitate is then indicated.[100] Four units of FFP contain the same amount of fibrinogen (about 2 grams) and Factor VIII (1000 units) as 10 units of cryoprecipitate. The choice of component then depends upon volume constraints (not usually a concern in the massively transfused patient) and whether Factor V or other clotting factor replacement is indicated.

Diffuse or intractable bleeding early after adequate surgical hemostasis has been achieved may be due to thrombocytopenia rather than to dilution of coagulation factors. In such bleeding patients, administration of platelet concentrate is indicated to maintain a platelet count of 50×10^9/L. Ten units of platelet concentrates contain as much as 500 mL of plasma, which has the same amount of stable coagulation factors as two units of fresh frozen plasma.

Patients who continue to bleed despite adequate levels of platelets and/or coagulation factors should be considered for surgical exploration. Close communication between the clinicians and the transfusion service director is mandatory in these situations.

25

Obstetrical Transfusion Practices and Hemolytic Disease of the Newborn

Fetal red blood cells contain blood group antigens inherited from the father that may be lacking in the mother. Due to fetal-maternal hemorrhage, a small percentage of mothers make blood group antibodies against these paternally derived antigens before or after birth of their offspring. Maternal IgG antibodies are transported across the placenta and can cause hemolysis of fetal red blood cells. This syndrome, hemolytic disease of the newborn (HDN), can vary in severity from hydropic death in utero to only IgG sensitization of fetal red blood cells without apparent hemolysis.

The most common cause of clinically significant HDN is the anti-D antibody. The incidence of Rh HDN is declining, however, due to the use of antenatal RhIG, as well as the additional prophylaxis with RhIG provided at delivery for Rh-negative mothers with Rh-positive infants.[77,78] Clinically significant HDN due to ABO incompatibility between mother and fetus is rare, although this serological situation occurs frequently. Many other blood groups, such as Kell and Duffy, as well as other Rh system antigens such as c, can cause immunization in both Rh-positive and Rh-negative women.

Antibody screening of obstetrical patients identifies those women with blood group antibodies capable of causing HDN. Pregnant women should have an ABO and Rh type and an antibody screen performed at an early prenatal visit. If the antibody screen is negative, additional antibody screening at 24-28 weeks of gestation is recommended.

If antibody is detected, the specificity should be determined and titers performed if the antibody is associated with HDN. IgG antibodies such as anti-D, anti-c and anti-E are likely to cause hemolytic disease. IgM, cold-reactive antibodies (eg, anti-I, anti-Le^a and anti-P$_1$) do not cause HDN because IgM antibodies do not cross the placenta.

Intrauterine Transfusion

A fetus severely affected with HDN (as determined by amniocentesis or ultrasonography) and too premature to deliver requires intrauterine transfusion. It is seldom feasible before

24-26 weeks' gestation. Blood for transfusion should be serologically compatible with the mother's serum. Group O Rh-negative red blood cells, negative for the antigen corresponding to the maternal antibody, are used for all intrauterine transfusions. Washed or deglycerolized red blood cells are usually selected to minimize the chance of transfusing incompatible alloagglutinins to a fetus of unknown ABO group. This technique also reduces the number of leukocytes transfused into the fetus. The desired hematocrit of the red blood cell component depends on the technique used and should be designed to reduce the risk of volume overload in the fetus. The volume transfused is determined according to the gestational age and approximation of blood volume.

A technique for intravascular transfusion performed in utero involving percutaneous umbilical blood sampling (PUBS) has been described. It avoids fetoscopy, permits estimation of hematocrit and is performed with continuous ultrasound visualization.[101] Once transfusions are initiated they should be continued every 10-21 days, depending on the clinical situation, until the infant is viable. Blood for intrauterine transfusion and subsequent exchange transfusion should be irradiated (1500-5000 rad) to avoid the rare complication of GVHD in the infant.

Exchange Transfusion

While hemolytic disease due to ABO incompatibility is usually so mild that exchange transfusion is rarely required, infants affected by hemolysis due to anti-D antibodies may require several exchange transfusions. The blood chosen should be compatible with the mother's serum and ABO group-compatible with the infant. Blood less than 7 days old is usually used in order to ensure maximum red cell viability and avoid low pH, decreased red cell 2,3-DPG and high plasma potassium levels. A final hematocrit of 0.50-0.60 (50-60%) in the component used for exchange is desirable.

Prevention of CMV Disease Transmission

Blood components should be processed or selected to reduce the risk of CMV disease in high risk infants, particularly in geographic areas where posttransfusion CMV transmission is a problem (see Pediatric Transfusion Practices).

26

Pediatric Transfusion Practices

Transfusion

Anemia in newborns may result from red cell loss due to the multiple blood sampling needed for laboratory testing or from pathological bleeding. The relatively slow rate with which the newborn bone marrow responds may also prolong the duration of anemia. Newborns require transfusions more frequently than older children, accounting for up to one-third of transfusions in one pediatric hospital.[102] Mean exposure can be 10-20 donors for each infant.

The indications for transfusion in the neonate varies from that of the adult as a result of the infant's physiologic immaturity, small blood volume and inability to tolerate minimal stress. The decision to transfuse is usually based on multiple parameters including calculated blood loss over a given time period, expected hemoglobin levels and clinical status (dyspnea, apnea, respiratory distress, poor weight gain). The transfusion of 10 mL/kg of red blood cells over a 2-3 hour period should raise the hemoglobin concentration by approximately 30 g/L (3 g/dL).

Transfusion services providing blood for neonates have developed methods of preparing 50-140 mL pediatric units of whole blood or red blood cells. This practice can decrease blood wastage associated with requests for small volume transfusions, and reduce donor exposure for those infants who are maintained with transfusions from the same unit for several days. Usually group O Rh-positive and/or negative blood is prepared in this fashion and therefore available for any pediatric patient.

''Walking donors,'' usually individuals working in neonatal nurseries who donate small samples of blood drawn into heparinized syringes, are not acceptable. Hepatitis and HIV testing, compatibility testing, using the correct amount of heparin, and careful record-keeping are not always possible with this program and the risks involved with transfusion may be needlessly increased.

Compatibility testing must be performed before the initial transfusion. Maternal serum can be used for testing neonatal (under 4 months) recipients since IgG blood group antibodies are passively transferred from mother to infant during gestation. For older infants (over 4 months) and children, samples for compatibility testing are obtained from the patient. Since infants less than 4 months old rarely produce antibodies against blood group antigens,[103] patients within this age group do not require repeated compatibility testing provided the initial antibody screen is negative and the red cells used for transfusion are either group O or an ABO type the same as or compatible with both the mother and child.

Blood used for transfusion should have adequate amounts of 2,3-DPG to ensure optimal delivery of oxygen to the tissues. Blood less than 7 days old is often selected for this purpose. Such units also have relatively low plasma potassium levels.

CMV-Negative Blood

Premature infants who are born to mothers who are CMV antibody negative or of unknown serologic status, and who weigh less than 1200 g at birth, may be at increased risk of morbidity and mortality from transfusion-transmitted CMV. Accordingly, for these or other high risk patients, it is prudent to provide blood from CMV-seronegative donors. Deglycerolized red blood cells, which are depleted of leukocytes, appear to be safe for transfusing these patients as well.[104,105]

Irradiated Blood

Graft-vs-host disease (GVHD) has been reported in pediatric patients with congenital or acquired immunodeficiency and infants following intrauterine exchange transfusion. Gamma irradiation of cellular blood components is effective in preventing GVHD in patients who are at high risk of developing this complication.[106]

27

Management of Alloimmunization

The refractory state to platelet transfusion, which usually accompanies alloimmunization, is one of the most serious and difficult to manage of all transfusion hazards.[13,107] Most of the clinically relevant antiplatelet antibodies bind to HLA antigens. Since a random platelet donor has a very small (<1:1000) chance of being HLA-matched with the recipient,[108] a patient who is extensively alloimmunized is very unlikely to have a good response to transfusion of platelets from random donors.

Ideally, in this situation, HLA-matched donors are identified and used to provide compatible apheresis platelets to the alloimmunized recipient. The use of HLA-matched platelets should restore responsiveness to platelet transfusion and eliminate febrile reactions.[17] This ideal management is difficult to achieve in practice, for a variety of reasons. The most common problem is that a sufficient number of HLA-matched donors may not be available to provide continuous support. While family members are more likely to be well-matched for HLA antigens, they may not be locally available, may not be eligible as donors or may be avoided due to their potential as bone marrow donors. This may be partially ameliorated by providing platelets from donors who have one or more HLA antigens that are not matched with the recipient but which are known to be included in antigen groups that are cross-reactive with those of the recipient.[109] This "selective HLA mismatching" technique significantly diminishes the size of the donor pool required to identify candidate donors. Selective HLA mismatching is effective in some, but not most, refractory patients and transfusion occurrences, owing chiefly to the difficulty in obtaining a good match grade.[110]

In some cases even the use of platelets that are well-matched for HLA antigens do not result in an adequate 1-hour platelet recovery (see p. 12). This may be due to a number of complicating factors, including splenomegaly, platelet consumption[21] and platelet ABO incompatibility.[111] In addition, it has been reported that the presence of non-HLA platelet alloantibodies may limit the response to HLA-matched platelets.[18,107] In response to this problem, experimental platelet crossmatching techniques have been developed and are reported to be effective in identifying donors whose platelets are more likely to have good posttransfusion recovery[18,112]; however, these techniques are still investigational and are available in only a few blood centers. Other methods of circumventing alloimmunization, such as the use of high dose intravenous immunoglobulin, anti-D (in Rh-positive patients), plasmapheresis or splenectomy have met with marginal success.[113]

Decisions regarding the use of HLA-matched, selectively mismatched or crossmatched platelets depend on several factors, including the availability of family members (and their potential as bone marrow donors), the availability of a sufficiently large pool of HLA-matched or selectively mismatched donors, and local access to a research lab that performs platelet crossmatching. In view of the complexity and difficulty of managing the hemotherapy of alloimmunized patients, all patients who are refractory to platelet transfusions should be managed in close cooperation with the transfusion service physician. Finally, the prevention of alloimmunization is a major goal. Recent clinical studies suggest that the incidence of alloimmunization may be decreased by exclusive transfusion of leukocyte-poor blood components produced by new filtration methods.

Transplantation

The goal of transfusion therapy in transplant patients is the appropriate replacement of deficient components without any deleterious effects on the graft. The approach will in part depend on the type of transplantation to be performed.

Evidence indicates that transfusions prior to bone marrow transplantation are deleterious.[114] Blood components from the donor or immediate family must be avoided, and for patients with aplastic anemia, exposure to all blood components prior to transplantation must be minimized. Leukocyte-poor RBC and platelet components are useful in such patients. In contrast, preoperative (and to a lesser extent, perioperative) transfusion enhances renal allograft survival. With living related donors, pretreatment with blood from the prospective kidney donor is a practical alternative to random transfusions.[115] Early evidence supports the use of preoperative blood transfusion even in cyclosporine-treated patients.[116] While alloimmunization to major histocompatibility complex antigens is not a major consideration when providing blood component support in potential liver transplant patients, concern centers around the large volumes of RBCs, FFP, cryoprecipitate and platelets that are required during liver transplantation.

GVHD is a major complication of bone marrow transplantation. Patients with allogeneic bone marrow transplants should receive components that contain viable lymphocytes, irradiated prior to transfusion, for an indefinite time after transplantation. Autologous bone marrow transplant patients also require irradiated components as long as their cell-mediated immunity remains abnormal posttransplant.

Serologic problems can result from major and minor incompatibilities between the donor and the recipient. Recipient production of antibody against donor red cell antigens or passenger donor lymphocyte production of antibody against recipient red cell antigens can result in delayed or acute hemolysis following bone marrow or kidney transplantation. Passive transfer of red cell antibodies has occurred with intravenous gammaglobulin or antilymphoblast globulin.

Blood and component support should be selected or processed to reduce the risk of CMV transmission in seronegative recipients who are likely to receive a seronegative graft.

Therapeutic Apheresis

Description

Therapeutic apheresis is the separation and removal of that portion of a patient's blood that contains a putative pathogenic component. While each manual plasmapheresis can remove 200-600 mL of plasma, a plasma exchange of several liters (usually at least one plasma volume) is better performed utilizing a machine that can separate, collect and reinfuse the various blood fractions. Most plasma exchange regimens include six procedures over 10-14 days. The large amount of plasma removed must be replaced with colloid or crystalloid solutions. Cytapheresis includes procedures that remove platelets, lymphocytes, granulocytes or erythrocytes. Centrifugal separation machines can be used for plasma exchange and cytapheresis. Plasma exchange alone can also be performed using membrane filtration technology, which can efficiently separate cell-free plasma from whole blood.[117]

Indications

Cytapheresis

Red blood cell exchange has been successful in elevating the levels of Hb A greater than 50% and has been reported useful in managing complications of sickle cell disease. These include recurrent stroke, priapism, ankle ulcers, obstetrical complications and sustained sickle cell crisis, unresponsive to standard therapy. Control studies have not been reported.[118] Therapeutic leukapheresis to treat leukostasis in acute myeloid leukemia or chronic granulocytic leukemia in blast crisis has been performed. The problem frequently occurs when most of the cells present are immature blasts or promyelocytes. Selection of patients for leukapheresis as an adjunct to chemotherapy depends on the clinical setting. When used it can transiently lower white blood cell counts. Effective chemotherapy should be instituted as soon as possible since leukapheresis is of short-term benefit. In patients with malignant platelet disorders and a risk of thrombosis and hemorrhage (platelet count greater than 1000×10^9/L), platelet pheresis may be useful until chemotherapy is effective.

Photopheresis

A special apheresis technique called photopheresis has been found efficacious for cutaneous T-cell lymphoma/leukemia (CTCL).[119] The technique requires patient ingestion of the drug psoralen several hours prior to the procedure. Psoralen binds to DNA in all nucleated cells, and upon stimulation with ultraviolet light, prevents DNA replication. After psoralen ingestion, a leukapheresis is performed and the white cells are continuously exposed to ultraviolet light before being returned to the patient. Active research using this technique in a variety of immunologic diseases is underway.

Plasma Exchange

Diseases that have clearly shown benefit from plasma exchange include hyperviscosity syndrome associated with hyperglobulinemia, acute myasthenia gravis, Guillain-Barré syndrome, chronic relapsing inflammatory polyneuropathy, Goodpasture's syndrome, cryoglobulinemia and thrombotic thrombocytopenic purpura (TTP). Plasmapheresis, although reported to be of value, is considered experimental for many other diseases. Often, only a clinical change in patient status can be monitored, since no specific laboratory test is available. More research is needed to establish indications and efficacy. Some recent review articles provide a thorough discussion of the indications for apheresis.[120,121]

Vascular Access

Vascular access is frequently a problem in apheresis patients. Antecubital veins are preferred but may be too small in some patients. Fistulas, grafts or shunts are ready sites of vascular access for apheresis. If a central venous catheter is used for apheresis, caution is required during rapid reinfusion of citrated blood, since the citrate may depress ionized calcium levels and lead to cardiac arrhythmias. Femoral vein catheters can be used but patients require close observation for hemorrhage after the procedure is terminated. Multi-lumen catheters are being used more frequently to provide vascular access since multiple procedures are performed during a course of therapy. Peripheral leg veins have an increased risk of thrombosis and should be avoided if possible.

Special Considerations

Albumin, saline or a combination of the two are often used as replacement solutions.[122] Use of FFP for fluid replacement is rarely indicated due to the risk of transfusion-transmitted diseases. However, it is the replacement solution of choice in patients with TTP and may be indicated for replacing coagulation factors if repeated daily procedures are required. Hypotension, paresthesia, volume overload and vasovagal reactions can occur during the procedure. Rare reactions include cardiac arrhythmia, cardiac arrest, respiratory arrest, anaphylaxis associated with fresh frozen plasma infusions, seizures and even death.[122] Long-term effects of apheresis are unknown.

The most critical step in preparing for transfusion is correctly identifying the patient and labeling the blood sample at the bedside. After blood collection, the wristband and labels should be checked and the appropriate forms signed and dated.

At the time of transfusion, the blood component with the compatibility tag attached must be compared with the patient's wristband at the bedside. Complete and careful identification is essential. No discrepancies in spelling or identification numbers should exist. The patient should remain under direct observation for 5-10 minutes after the infusion begins and must be checked periodically until the transfusion is completed.

Blood Warming

Transfusion of cold blood at rates over 100 mL/minute has been associated with a high rate of cardiac arrest when compared to a control group receiving warm blood.[123] There is no evidence that patients receiving 1-3 units of blood slowly over several hours receive additional benefit from blood warming.

Blood warmers are of two types: 1) a coil of plastic tubing placed in a temperature-monitored waterbath at no more than 38 C and 2) electrically heated plates in contact with a flat plastic blood bag. Automatic warming devices must have a visible thermometer and should have an audible warning system, since thermal red cell injury occurs at temperatures over 40 C. Warming the whole unit of blood by immersion in hot water or by the use of microwave blood warmers is not recommended, since hemolysis can be caused by overheating.[124]

The use of blood warmers is generally restricted to:

1. Adult patients receiving rapid and multiple transfusions (rate over 50 mL/kg/hour).
2. Exchange transfusions in infants.
3. Children receiving large volumes (over 15 mL/kg/hour).
4. Patients with cold agglutinins active in vitro at 37 C.
5. Rapid infusion through central venous catheters.

Time Limits for Infusing Blood Components

A unit of blood should not be kept at room temperature for more than a short time due to the risk of bacterial growth. If clinical conditions require an infusion time of greater than 4 hours, the unit should be divided into aliquots and portions kept in the blood bank refrigerator until required. Changing of the blood filter every 4 hours is also recommended. A unit of blood that has been allowed to warm above 10 C, but not used, cannot be reissued by the transfusion service. Blood must never be stored in unmonitored refrigerators.

Concomitant Use of Intravenous Solutions

Only normal saline (0.9% USP) may be administered with blood components. Other solutions may be hypotonic (eg, 5% dextrose in water) and cause hemolysis in vitro, or contain additives such as calcium (Ringer's lactate) that can initiate in vitro coagulation in citrated blood.[125] To increase infusion rate and decrease viscosity, red blood cells may be diluted with normal saline (0.9% USP); single-donor or FFP plasma can be used, if indicated, but this increases the risk of transfusion-transmitted diseases. Normal serum albumin (5%) is acceptable in special circumstances. Medications should never be added to a unit of blood because: 1) some drugs may cause hemolysis due to their excessively high pH; 2) if a drug is added to blood and subsequently the unit is discontinued due to a transfusion reaction, the dose of the drug infused may not be known; 3) if the drug is added to blood it would be difficult to decide if any adverse reactions were due to the drug or to the blood.

Filters

All blood components must be administered through a filter to remove blood clots and other debris. Standard 170-micron blood filters trap large macroaggregates, but not the microaggregates that form progressively in blood after 5 days of storage. These microaggregates can lodge in the pulmonary circulation but their role in the development of pulmonary toxicity is unproven.[126] Microaggregate blood filters of 20-40 micron pore size can remove more of this microaggregate debris, but they are not indicated for routine (1-2 unit) blood transfusions. A lack of benefit for use of the filters has been shown for patients requiring an average 7 units of blood for elective surgical procedures.[127] The use of microaggregate filters should be restricted to patients transfused during cardio-pulmonary bypass (where the microaggregates enter the systemic circulation directly) and the setting of massive transfusion. Disadvantages include potential for becoming clogged and resistance to rapid blood delivery. Special filters are presently available to provide leukocyte-poor components (see p. 15).

Transfusion of Platelets and Granulocytes

Platelets and granulocytes are routinely administered through a standard blood filter administration set at a rate of 1-2 mL/minute or as tolerated by the patient. Pediatric patients requiring platelet or granulocyte transfusions may require concentrates with decreased plasma volumes. Patients with a history of recurrent febrile reactions to these components may benefit from premedication with antipyretics other than aspirin (see p. 11). Leukocyte removal filters can be used for transfusion of platelets in such patients. Corticosteroids may be helpful in patients with severe reactions. Subcutaneous or intravenous meperidine can control the severe shaking chill reactions sometimes seen with granulocyte or platelet infusions.

Infusion Devices

A variety of electronic infusion devices or "blood pumps" are available. These machines are designed to deliver parenteral fluids, including blood components, at flow rates as low as 1 mL/hour. The pump mechanisms vary with different manufacturers and include syringe-type pumping systems, peristaltic roller devices and electromechanical pumps, which operate on a positive volumetric displacement principle.

Some systems require manufacturer-supplied pump cassettes, while others can be used with standard intravenous administration set tubing. Although most pump systems do not induce mechanical hemolysis when used with whole blood, gross hemolysis may result when some models are used to administer red blood cells. This is attributable to the high shear forces generated with use of high hematocrit red cell concentrates, which are quite viscous. Available data show that use of the pumps with other blood components, such as platelets and granulocytes is acceptable.[128,129] If these pumps are to be used to administer units of red blood cells or other components, the manufacturer should be consulted regarding the suitability of the instrument for this purpose.

SECTION IV

HEMOSTATIC DISORDERS

Overview of Hemostasis

Hemostasis refers to the totality of processes concerned with the control of bleeding. Hemostasis is dependent upon distinct but interactive elements: blood vessels (particularly the endothelial layer), cellular blood elements (particularly platelets), plasma procoagulant proteins (clotting or coagulation factors) and two control processes, the fibrinolytic system and inhibitory or anticoagulant proteins. Pathologic bleeding or thrombosis may occur due to derangements in any of these elements.

Blood Vessels

The normal endothelium is maintained as a thromboresistant surface by a variety of mechanisms, including the production of the antiplatelet prostaglandin prostacyclin. After injury, subendothelial structures stimulate activation of the procoagulant elements of the system. Platelets adhere to subendothelium in seconds, followed minutes later by the elaboration of fibrin and formation of a platelet-fibrin clot.

Hereditary blood vessel disorders associated with a bleeding diathesis include disorders of vessel connective tissue structures, such as osteogenesis imperfecta, pseudoxanthoma elasticum and the Ehlers-Danlos and Marfan syndromes. Vascular malformations, which can cause recurrent bleeding, include telangiectasia (Osler-Weber-Rendu syndrome), angiodysplasia and giant hemangioma.

Acquired blood vessel disorders include scurvy and vasculitis. Treatment is directed to the underlying disease. Postoperative bleeding due to inadequate surgical hemostasis may be difficult to diagnose, particularly in patients with abnormalities of platelets or coagulation factors. When measurable, blood loss above 5 mL/kg/hour often indicates inadequate surgical hemostasis.[130]

Platelets

Platelets are anuclear cells that form a cohesive plug at vessel injury sites. This plug formation is called primary hemostasis.

Thrombocytopenia and platelet function defects are frequent causes of abnormal hemostasis. Platelet function is routinely assessed by two screening tests: the platelet count and the bleeding time. Bleeding risk increases as the platelet count falls below 100×10^9/L. In patients with underlying lesions or about to undergo invasive procedures, platelet transfusions are often indicated for counts less than 50×10^9/L.[100] In contrast, in nonbleeding patients without underlying lesions, such as the patient receiving chemotherapy, prophylactic platelet transfusions are usually given at counts below 20×10^9/L.

Platelet function defects are usually diagnosed by finding a prolonged bleeding time with a normal platelet count. A bleeding time of 15 minutes or above generally signifies an increased bleeding risk.[131,132]

Platelets serve an important role in the coagulation system as well, by storage of coagulation proteins within platelet granules and through special platelet membrane receptors, which form a reaction surface for coagulation factor interactions.

Coagulation Proteins

The coagulation mechanism consists of a closely regulated series of reactions culminating in the formation of an insoluble protein gel called fibrin. The initial platelet plug is covered with fibrin strands, stabilizing the clot. The system consists of: procoagulant serine proteases that circulate as zymogens (Factors II, VII, IX, X, XI, XII, prekallikrein), nonenzymatic cofactors (Factors V, VIII, kininogen), fibrinogen, the substrate for the fibrin gel, and a fibrin stabilizing enzyme, Factor XIII. Surfaces, which include endothelium and platelet membranes, and calcium ions are required during most of the reactions.

Screening tests of coagulation include the prothrombin time (PT, evaluates Factors II, V, VII, X), the partial thromboplastin time (PTT, evaluates Factors II, V, VIII, IX, XII, prekallikrein, kininogen), the thrombin time (TT, evaluates the fibrinogen-to- fibrin conversion step) and a quantitative fibrinogen assay. Mild-to-moderate prolongations of PT, PTT and TT are not often associated with significant decreases in coagulation factor levels or with increased bleeding risk.[100,133] The therapeutic levels of these factors required for hemostasis and the indications for factor replacement depend upon the patient's clinical status (see p. 22, Table 3). In general, factor levels above 20-30% and fibrinogen levels above 1 g/L (100 mg/dL) are sufficient to prevent major hemorrhage.[100]

Both congenital and acquired disorders of coagulation are common. Common congenital disorders include von Willebrand's disease and hemophilia, while liver disease and consumptive disorders due to trauma, shock or infection are common acquired disorders. When possible, significant disorders of coagulation should be treated in consultation with a hematologist.

Fibrinolysis and Other Control Mechanisms of Hemostasis

The process by which procoagulant activities are limited to the site of injury and the repair is initiated, are important regulators of normal hemostasis. Two main processes are involved: the inhibitory system, consisting primarily of circulating and endothelial-based protease inhibitors, and the fibrinolytic system, responsible for the proteolytic dissolution of the fibrin clot. Inhibitory proteins include antithrombin III, with broad specificity against procoagulant serine proteases, and alpha-2-macroglobulin. Two anticoagulant serine proteases, protein C and protein S, provide feedback control of coagulation by proteolysis of Factors V and VIII. Deficiencies of antithrombin III and proteins C and S can lead to pathologic thrombosis.

Fibrinolysis is accomplished by the enzyme plasmin, formed by the action of endothelial-based activators upon its circulating zymogen, plasminogen. Plasminogen and its activators bind to the forming fibrin clot, providing the mechanisms for local clot dissolution from within. Plasmin's natural plasma inhibitor, alpha-2-plasmin inhibitor, plays an important physiologic role, since a deficiency leads to unchecked plasmin action and a bleeding disorder. Plasmin has other anticoagulant activity as well, including the proteolysis of Factors V, VIII and fibrinogen and alteration of platelet membrane receptors.

The laboratory hallmark of an activated fibrinolytic system is detection of free plasmin in the blood. No direct assay is available; instead, any of several tests may be utilized. These include a fall in the plasma fibrinogen, plasminogen or alpha-2-inhibitor levels or an elevation in the TT or PTT. Fibrin(ogen) degradation products (FDPs) produced by plasmin action can inhibit fibrin formation and impair platelet function.

Platelet Disorders

A wide variety of conditions can result in thrombocytopenia. Bone marrow suppression or destruction, as seen with radiation, chemotherapy, some infections and toxic drugs or chemicals, are the most common causes. In this situation, platelet transfusions are usually successful in elevating the platelet count and lowering bleeding risk. Accelerated destruction of peripheral blood platelets, as seen with sepsis, consumptive or immune disorders, are more difficult to treat with transfusions, since the transfused platelets are also rapidly destroyed. Platelet transfusions are generally not indicated in autoimmune or alloimmune thrombocytopenia, since survival of the transfused platelets is very brief.[130]

Platelet function defects may be congenital or acquired. Congenital disorders include abnormalities of platelet granules or membrane receptors. Acquired disorders are most often caused by drugs, especially aspirin and other nonsteroidal anti-inflammatory agents. Patients with uremia and patients undergoing procedures utilizing extracorporeal circulation often have platelet function defects.[131,132] Platelet transfusion can be used to treat selected platelet function defects; however, repeated transfusions may result in alloimmunization and therapeutic ineffectiveness. Recently, successful shortening of prolonged bleeding times, with cessation of bleeding, has been obtained using desmopressin (1-deamino-8-D-arginine vasopressin, DDAVP). Desmopressin releases Factor VIII, von Willebrand factor (vWF) and plasminogen activator from endothelial cells and other storage sites. The mechanism of action in the improvement in platelet function is unclear, but may relate to elevated levels of the adhesive protein, vWF. Desmopressin has been reported to be effective in treating bleeding in uremia, reducing blood loss during cardiopulmonary bypes and in congenital platelet function abnormalities.[134] Desmopressin is usually given at doses of 0.3 mg/kg over 20 minutes. Tachyphylaxis may develop with repeated doses, diminishing its effectiveness. Potential side effects include hypertension, fluid retention and allergic reactions.

Congenital Disorders of Coagulation

von Willebrand's Disease

von Willebrand's disease (vWD) is a common autosomal dominant trait characterized by abnormalities of von Willebrand factor (vWF), a large multimeric molecule that circulates in plasma bound to procoagulant factor VIII. vWF is necessary for platelet adhesion to subendothelial tissue; therefore, platelet plug formation is deficient in vWD. Factor VIII levels are also diminished, due to a low level of its carrier protein, vWF. vWD presents as a platelet function defect, and the diagnosis is confirmed by specific assays for vWF and Factor VIII. Most forms of mild or moderate vWD can be treated with desmopressin.[135] Desmopressin is contraindicated in the rare type IIb variant. Severe forms are treated with cryoprecipitate, which is enriched in vWF and Factor VIII. Most lyophilized Factor VIII concentrates do not contain therapeutic levels of vWF.

Hemophilia A—Factor VIII Deficiency

Hemophilia A results from a deficiency of Factor VIII caused by an X chromosome abnormality. vWF levels are normal. Patients with Factor VIII levels above 10 percent are considered mild hemophiliacs, and significant trauma usually precedes bleeding episodes. Moderate hemophiliacs have Factor VIII levels of 2-10% and bleed abnormally with minimal trauma. Severe hemophiliacs (Factor VIII levels less than 1-2%) are at risk for spontaneous hemorrhage.

Unlike platelet-related bleeding, hemophilic bleeding manifests several hours after the causative trauma and occurs frequently in deep structures, such as joints and muscles. However, bleeding may occur anywhere, including intracranially and in the gastrointestinal tract.

Mild or moderate hemophilia A may be treated with desmopressin,[135] whereas severe disease requires infusion of cryoprecipitate or lyophilized Factor VIII concentrates. Levels from 30-100%, depending upon the clinical condition, are achieved using the following formula:

Plasma volume (PV, mL) = 40 mL/kg × body weight (kg)
Factor VIII units infused = [(PV) × (% increase desired)]
divided by 100

When using cryoprecipitate, the number of Factor VIII units is divided by 80 to obtain the number of bags required. The Factor VIII activity of lyophilized concentrates appears on the container label. After therapeutic levels are achieved, transfusions are generally repeated every 8-12 hours (the half-life of Factor VIII) until healing occurs.

Hemophilia B—Factor IX Deficiency

The clinical manifestations of Factor IX deficiency are similar to those of Factor VIII deficiency. Desmopressin and cryoprecipitate are ineffective in treatment, however. Factor IX is replaced with plasma (fresh frozen or single donor) or lyophilized factor IX concentrates, which may contain Factors II, VII and X as well. Plasma contains 1 unit per mL of Factor IX activity, whereas the contents of the lyophilized material appear on the label. Factor IX has a half-life of 18-24 hours and posttransfusion recovery is half the predicted value, due to extravascular distribution. Therefore, some physicians compensate for this low recovery by doubling the dose suggested by the formula.

34

Acquired Disorders of Coagulation

Acquired Anticoagulants

In 10-15% of severe hemophiliacs, IgG antibodies to Factor VIII develop as an alloimmune response to repeated Factor VIII infusion.[60] Therapy must be individualized and always requires consultation with a hematologist, expert in the treatment of hemophiliacs.

Rarely, spontaneous Factor VIII inhibitors occur as an autoimmune process in previously normal individuals. Severe bleeding can occur. Inhibitors to other coagulation factors occur very rarely. Another acquired anticoagulant is the "lupus-type" inhibitor, usually an IgG reacting with a phospholipid component of the reaction surface. These inhibitors are not associated with bleeding unless Factor II levels are also diminished. Paradoxically, they may be associated with thrombotic disorders.

The laboratory hallmark of the inhibitors is the finding of a prolonged PT and/or PTT, depending upon the specificity of the inhibitor, which is not shortened when the test is repeated with a 1:1 mixture of patient and normal plasma.

Heparin may lead to noncorrectable prolongations in the PTT or TT. Heparin markedly enhances the ability of antithrombin III to neutralize serine proteases and is used as an anticoagulant in a wide variety of clinical situations. Even small amounts of heparin, eg, the flush volume in a subclavian catheter, can prolong the TT and PTT leading to confusion in diagnosis.

Vitamin K Deficiency and Antigonism: Vitamin K is a fat-soluble vitamin necessary for the synthesis in the liver of Factors II, VII, IX, X, protein C and protein S. Deficiency states occur in malnourished individuals who are receiving antibiotics and in patients with general fat malabsorption states, such as celiac disease, pancreatic insufficiency or obstructive jaundice. Administration of vitamin K corrects the deficiency state in 12-36 hours. Urgent correction can be accomplished by plasma transfusions. Oral anticoagulants, dicumarol and warfarin, work by antagonizing vitamin K dependent syntheses of the above factors. Warfarin overdose is treated by withdrawal of the drug and, if bleeding is severe, by plasma transfusion.

Liver Disease: Patients with liver disease have multiple hemostatic derangements, including coagulation factor deficiencies, impaired vitamin K utilization and activated fibrinolysis. Thrombocytopenia due to hypersplenism may be clinically significant. Treatment with plasma is indicated when bleeding is present, but prophylactic plasma infusions have limited clinical utility due to the short half-lives of the vitamin K dependent factors. Factor IX concentrates are not indicated due to increased risk of thromboembolic complications.

Disseminated Intravascular Coagulation (DIC): Free thrombin in the blood is the cause of DIC. Thrombin can be generated by pathologic release of thromboplastic substances into the blood or by widespread endothelial damage, leading to platelet and coagulation system activation. Common clinical conditions predisposing to DIC include sepsis, trauma, incomplete abortion, shock and malignancy. The resultant widespread intravascular clotting may lead to severe organ ischemia. Bleeding, due to consumption of platelets, fibrinogen and Factors II, V and VIII, may also occur. Diagnostic laboratory hallmarks are: thrombocytopenia, hypofibrinogenemia and elevated FDPs. Treatment is first aimed at the primary process. If ischemia is the prominent clinical finding, heparin may be infused to inhibit thrombin generation. Bleeding due to deficiency states can be corrected by platelet, plasma and/or cryoprecipitate infusions. Consultation with a hematologist should be obtained when possible, especially if heparin use is contemplated.

35

Disorders of Fibrinolysis and Other Control Mechanisms

Antithrombin III Deficiency: Antithrombin III potentiates the in vivo effect of heparin. Congenital deficiency states are associated with a thrombotic diathesis, even in patients with as much as 50% of normal levels. Replacement therapy with plasma or lyophilized AT-III concentrates should accompany heparin infusions when treating thrombosis.[82,136]

Alpha-2-Plasmin Inhibitor Deficiency: Deficiencies of alpha-2-plasmin inhibitor, the primary circulating plasmin inhibitor, are associated with a severe hemorrhagic disorder. As with AT-III deficiency, diagnosis requires a specific assay for this inhibitor. Therapy consists of replacement by plasma transfusion and/or oral antifibrinolytic agents such as epsilon aminocaproic acid (EACA).

Protein C and Protein S: Deficiencies of these two vitamin K dependent anticoagulant proteins are associated with recurrent thromboembolic disease and a purpura fulminant-type disorder. Diagnosis is established by specific assays. Protein C levels are diminished by oral anticoagulant therapy and by DIC. Therapy for congenitally deficient patients is provided by plasma infusions.

Disorders of Fibrinolysis

Primary disorders of fibrinolysis, so-called systemic hyperfibrinolytic states, are rare and hard to differentiate from DIC. Most fibrinolytic states are secondary to strong procoagulant stimuli. Antifibrinolytic therapy, eg, EACA, has been reported as successful in bleeding states associated with an activated fibrinolytic mechanism, such as cardiopulmonary bypass procedures and liver transplantation. However, by blocking clot lysis, thrombotic complications often occur, with disastrous clinical sequelae. EACA is useful as adjunct therapy with factor replacement in hemophilia, in particular during and after dental procedures. Use of EACA should never be undertaken without hematologic consultation.

The therapeutic administration of the plasminogen activators streptokinase, urokinase or recombinant tissue-type plasminogen activator (t-PA) has grown increasingly important in the treatment of thrombotic disease.[138,139] These agents may be used locally (ie, infused via angiographic control directly into the thrombosed area) or systemically, via peripheral vein. Successful results have been reported in deep-vein thrombosis, intraabdonimal thrombosis, thrombosis at the site of indwelling catheters, pulmonary embolism and in peripheral and coronary arterial occlusions. Contraindications to therapy include recent cranial trauma or known intracranial lesions and recent major surgery. Laboratory monitoring is not precise and treatment regimens are standardized for each agent. The lytic state can be monitored in various ways (see p. 69) and simple demonstration that a lytic state exists using any method usually suffices.

SECTION V

TRANSFUSION REACTIONS

36

Acute Transfusion Reactions

Transfusion of any blood component presents a substantial risk to the recipient. Adverse reactions may occur in as many as 10% of recipients. Since many of these reactions are not preventable, transfusion therapy should be preceded by careful analysis of the risks and benefits of the therapy. Only when the benefits clearly outweigh the risks should transfusion be prescribed. Patients must be advised of risks, benefits and alternatives to transfusion.

Although hemolytic transfusion reactions are the most serious and potentially life-threatening, febrile and allergic reactions make up the majority of immediate reactions. Hypervolemia is probably more common than suspected due to under-reporting. The seriousness and the signs and symptoms of clinical transfusion reactions vary greatly. The majority of life-threatening transfusion reactions occur early in the course of transfusion. Therefore, all patients should be carefully monitored during transfusion for untoward reactions, and any adverse signs and symptoms should be promptly investigated.

Acute Hemolytic Reactions

These reactions can be divided into acute intravascular hemolysis, most due to ABO incompatibility, and acute extravascular hemolysis, usually due to incompatibility involving other red cell antigens and IgG antibodies. Nearly all acute hemolytic reactions result from clerical errors, either in labeling the blood specimen, or in identifying the blood unit or the patient. Rarely, blood bank technical errors are responsible.

Acute hemolytic reactions occur after infusion of incompatible red blood cells. Infusion of incompatible plasma, which may occur with transfusion of the plasma contained in ABO-incompatible platelet concentrates, rarely causes severe reactions due to the in vivo dilution of the antibody in the recipient's blood volume. Of course, incompatible plasma may be a more serious concern in infants and young children because of the small blood volume.

A transfusion reaction due to ABO incompatibility is clinically the most dangerous type. This occurs because anti-A and anti-B readily activate complement to C9, causing intravascular hemolysis. An ABO-incompatible transfusion reaction may also be associated with activation of the coagulation system and release of vasoactive amines. These event can result in vasomotor instability, cardiorespiratory collapse or disseminated intravascular coagulation (DIC), any of which may be fatal. Renal damage may result from systemic hypotension, renal vasoconstriction and renovascular thrombi formation. The severity of the reaction is generally proportional to the amount of incompatible blood infused, the type of incompatibility, and the amount of time before treatment.

Acute extravascular hemolysis is usually seen with antibodies other than ABO, such as Kidd (Jk^a), Duffy (Fy^a) and Kell (K). Extravascular hemolysis is usually accompanied by fever, anemia, increase in bilirubin and development of a positive direct antiglobulin test. Severe clinical signs and symptoms are rare since activation of complement to C9 does not usually occur.

Febrile Reactions

Fever can be associated with many types of transfusion reactions, and may be the first sign of a serious hemolytic reaction. Febrile reactions, however, are usually attributable to antibodies (cytotoxic antibodies and leukoagglutinins) directed against leukocytes or platelets. This is a diagnosis of exclusion since definitive laboratory tests are not available. The reactions may begin with chills followed by a rise in temperature of 1.0 C (or over 38.3 C). These reactions can be prevented by transfusion of leukocyte-poor components.[6,31] The incidence of febrile transfusion reactions is low (1% of transfusions), and repeat reactions are uncommon.[32] Most febrile reactions will respond to antipyretic medication (aspirin or acetaminophen, see p. 11).

Allergic Reactions

These are probably caused by antibodies against plasma proteins. Signs and symptoms may vary from localized urticaria to systemic anaphylactic reactions. Urticarial reactions (hives, itching, erythema) occur in 1-2% of recipients. Nearly all reactions are mild, however, and respond to oral or intramuscular antihistamines. With mild urticarial reactions, the transfusion may be continued after antihistamines are administered, if symptoms subside.

Severe systemic reactions may require epinephrine and/or steroids. Rarely, severe reactions may be caused by IgG, anti-IgA antibodies in patients who are IgA deficient. Accordingly, patients with a history of anaphylactic transfusion reactions should be evaluated for the presence of anti-IgA antibody. If anti-IgA antibodies are found to be present, only extensively washed red blood cells and IgA-deficient plasma, obtainable from special donor depots, should be used for subsequent transfusion to these rare individuals.[141]

Hypervolemia

This problem results when either too much blood is given or it is infused too rapidly. Patients with chronic anemia are particularly at risk, since they are usually normovolemic. Except when treating active hemorrhage or acute hypovolemia, blood components should be infused slowly, with the infusion taking no more than 4 hours. Correction of the anemia over a period of days is preferable to rapid replacement with the resulting fluid overload producing cardiac failure. Signs of fluid overload include systolic hypertension (>50 mm rise), dyspnea and EKG abnormalities, notably premature ventricular contractions.

Noncardiogenic Pulmonary Edema

Leukocyte antibodies (anti-HLA or leukoagglutinins) may cause signs and symptoms of pulmonary edema with normal left ventricular filling pressures.[142,143] Antibody in the donor plasma, directed against antigens in the recipient, as well as antibody in the recipient directed against donor leukocytes have been implicated.[144] The reaction is probably unsuspected in many instances, but if recognized, should be reported to the blood bank for investigation. Fresh frozen plasma infusion has been implicated in this syndrome as well.[47]

Nonimmune Hemolysis

Erythrocytes may be hemolyzed by exposure to hypotonic solutions (5% dextrose in water), hypertonic solutions (50% dextrose in water), mechanical stress (cardiopulmonary bypass), improper storage (freezing or overheating) or, rarely, bacterial contamination. The cause of hemoglobinemia and/or hemoglobinuria must be evaluated as soon as possible since delay in the recognition of an immune hemolytic transfusion reaction could lead to serious clinical complications. Steps to identify and eliminate the cause of nonimmune hemolysis must be vigorously pursued.

Bacterial Sepsis

Bacterial sepsis, although a rare complication, has been reported due to red blood cell transfusion[145-147] and more recently, due to platelet concentrates.[148,149] Signs of sepsis will occur shortly after starting transfusion of a contaminated unit.

Investigation of Suspected Hemolytic Reactions

The following steps should be taken when a hemolytic reaction is suspected:

1. STOP TRANSFUSION. Keep IV patent with normal saline.
2. Notify attending physician and blood bank immediately.
3. Check blood bag compatibility tag, label and patient identification for clerical errors.
4. Send anticoagulated and clotted posttransfusion blood samples, properly labeled, and transfusion reaction form to the blood bank for investigation for hemoglobinemia and serologic incompatibility.
5. Send blood bag and freshly collected urine to the blood bank, if requested, for detection of bacterial contamination or hemoglobinuria, respectively.
6. If a hemolytic reaction is suspected or confirmed, obtain baseline BUN, creatinine and coagulation studies.

Treatment

Treatment depends on the type of reaction, as outlined in Table 5. Acute intravascular hemolysis is clinically more severe than extravascular hemolysis and must be treated vigorously. If an acute intravascular hemolytic reaction is suspected, the transfusion should be stopped and diuresis initiated as soon as possible. Fluid should be administered to maintain urine flow at 1-2 mL/kg/hour and to support the blood pressure. Furosemide or mannitol may be indicated. Low dose dopamine (<5 µg/kg/min) may also be required.[150] Coagulation parameters should be monitored for the development of DIC, which may require treatment with heparin and/or compatible blood components. If oliguria or anuria occurs, treatment for acute renal failure should be instituted.

Febrile reactions generally respond to antipyretics such as acetaminophen. Rarely, treatment of febrile reactions will require steroids. Leukocyte-poor red blood cells and/or platelets may be useful in preventing repeated reactions. Mild urticarial reactions can be treated with antihistamines and the transfusion continued. Severe systemic allergic reactions may require epinephrine or steroids.

Noncardiogenic pulmonary edema will require respiratory support and may benefit from the administration of fluids and/or steroids. Treatment of transfusion-induced hypervolemia is the same as that used for treatment of any fluid overload condition. Bacterial contamination and sepsis must be treated promptly with circulatory support and antibiotics.

Table 5. Transfusion Reactions

Type	Signs and Symptoms	Usual Cause	Treatment	Prevention
Acute intravascular hemolytic (immune)	Hemoglobinemia and hemoglobinuria, fever, chills, anxiety, shock, DIC, dyspnea, chest pain, flank pain	Incompatibility due to clerical errors, involves ABO (primarily) or other erythrocyte Ag-Ab incompatibility	Stop transfusion; hydrate, support blood pressure and respiration; induce diuresis; treat shock and DIC	Avoid clerical errors; insure proper sample and recipient identification
Delayed extravascular hemolytic (immune)	Fever, malaise, indirect hyperbilirubinemia, increased urine urobilinogen, falling hematocrit	Usually involves non-ABO Ag-Ab incompatibility occurring 3-10 days posttransfusion	Monitor hematocrit, renal function, coagulation profile; no acute treatment generally required	Avoid clerical errors
Febrile	Fever, chills, rarely hypotension	Antibodies to leukocytes or plasma proteins	Stop transfusion; give antipyretics: acetaminophen (or aspirin if not thrombocytopenic)	Pretransfusion antipyretic; leukocyte-poor blood components

Allergic	Urticaria (hives), rarely hypotension or anaphylaxis	Antibodies to plasma proteins	Stop transfusion; give antihistamine (PO or IM); if severe, epinephrine and/or steroids	Pretransfusion antihistamine; washed red cell components
Hypervolemic	Dyspnea, hypertension, pulmonary edema, cardiac arrhythmias	Too rapid and/or excessive blood transfusion	Induce diuresis; phlebotomy; support cardiorespiratory system as needed	Avoid rapid or excessive transfusion
Noncardiogenic pulmonary edema	Dyspnea, pulmonary edema, normal cardiac pressures	Anti-HLA or anti-leukocyte antibodies	Support blood pressure and respiration (may require intubation)	Washed red blood cells, avoid unnecessary transfusion
Bacterial sepsis	Shock, chills, fever	Contaminated blood component	Stop transfusion; support blood pressure; give antibiotics	Care in blood collection and storage

Delayed Transfusion Reactions

Delayed Hemolytic Reactions

These reactions are caused by the rapid production of red blood cell antibody shortly after transfusion of the corresponding antigen. The immune system may have been stimulated by previous transfusion, followed by a subsequent decrease in antibody to levels undetectable by routine compatibility testing methods. With the additional infusion of blood containing the antigen, an anamnestic response of antibody production occurs in 3-10 days, and the transfused red blood cells are destroyed, generally by extravascular hemolysis in the spleen. Complement may be activated, but usually stops at the level of C3. Delayed reactions may also occur after primary exposure to a foreign red cell antigen. It has been estimated that there is a 1-1.6% risk of sensitizing a recipient to a red cell antigen other than D with each unit of blood transfused.[151] Most patients will develop fever and anemia, and in some individuals, icterus due to indirect hyperbilirubinemia may be noted. Generally, no acute treatment is required. Rarely, however, hemolysis may be brisk enough to cause shock, renal failure and even death. These severe reactions, which usually include some degree of intravascular hemolysis, should be managed as outlined under treatment of acute hemolytic reactions.

Infectious Diseases

Many infections can be transmitted by blood transfusion. The most common disease causing serious clinical problems is hepatitis.[152] Posttransfusion hepatitis B occurs even though all donor blood is currently tested for HBsAg using sensitive techniques.[153] However, 90% of posttransfusion hepatitis is due to non-A,non-B (NANB) hepatitis. No specific test is available to detect NANB hepatitis. Surrogate testing for anti-HBc and alanine aminotransferase (ALT) is now performed on all donor blood and may reduce the risk of NANB hepatitis to 1% per unit transfused.[154] A test for NANB hepatitis, now called hepatitis C, is on the horizon. If posttransfusion hepatitis develops, the transfusion service most be notified, and the donors investigated. AIDS can be transmitted by blood transfusion.[155,156] Currently, all donors are tested for antibody to HIV. This test reduces the risk of HIV transmission by blood transfusion to a very low level (approximately 1:40,000 to 1:1,000,000 per blood component exposure). Efforts are regularly made to exclude donors who belong to known high risk groups. Donor blood is also tested for antibodies to HTLV-I. Epstein-Barr virus (EBV), CMV,[157] malaria[158] or toxoplasmosis[159] may also be transmitted by transfusion.

Other Delayed Reactions

Following frequent transfusions, alloimmunization to red cell, platelet and leukocyte (HLA) antigens may occur, resulting in crossmatching difficulty, febrile and allergic reactions and refractoriness to platelet transfusions. Chronic red cell transfusion in time results in iron overload hemosiderosis. Treatment with deferoxamine, an iron-chelating agent,[160] may reduce damage to the liver and heart.

Graft-vs-host disease may develop in patients with congenital immune deficiencies involving T lymphocytes as well as in recipients of allogeneic and autologous bone marrow grafts.[161] All cellular blood components given to such patients should be gamma irradiated.[106] Other groups considered to be at less risk for GVHD include infants receiving intrauterine and exchange transfusions and patients receiving immunosuppressive therapy for lymphoma and acute leukemia.

REFERENCES AND

READINGS

References

1. Holland PV, ed. Standards for blood banks and transfusion services, 13th ed. Arlington, VA: American Association of Blood Banks, 1989.

2. Moore GL, Ledford ME, Peck CC. The in vitro evaluation of modifications in CPD-adenine anticoagulated-preserved blood at various hematocrits. Transfusion 1980;20:419-26.

3. Walker RH. Special Report: Transfusion risks. Am J Clin Pathol 1987;88:374-8.

4. Heaton A, Miripol J, Aster R, et al. Use of Adsol preservation solution for prolonged storage of low viscosity AS-1 red blood cells. Br J Haematol 1984;57:467-78.

5. Simon TL, Marcus CS, Myhre BA, Nelson EJ. Effects of AS-3 nutrient-additive solution on 42 and 49 days of storage of red cells. Transfusion 1987;27:178-82.

6. Meryman HT, Hornblower M. The preparation of red cells depleted of leukocytes. Transfusion 1986;26:101-6.

7. Haugen RK. Hepatitis after the transfusion of frozen red cells and washed red cells. N Engl J Med 1979;301:393-5.

8. Chaplin H. Frozen red cells revisited. N Engl J Med 1984;311:1696-8.

9. Opelz G, Terasaki PI. Dominant effect of transfusion on kidney graft survival. Transplantation 1980;29:153-8.

10. Adler SP, Lawrence LT, Baggett J, Biro V, Sharp DE. Prevention of posttransfusion-associated cytomegalovirus infection in very low-birthweight infants using frozen blood and donors seronegative for cytomegalovirus. Transfusion 1984;24:333-5.

11. Murphy S, Kahn RA, Holme S, et al. Improved storage of platelets for transfusion in a new container. Blood 1982;60:1940200.

12. Schiffer CA, Lee EJ, Ness PM, Reilly J. Clinical evaluation of platelets stored for one to five days. Blood 1986;67:1591-4.

13. National Institute of Health Consensus development conference: Platelet transfusion therapy. JAMA 1987;257:1777-80.

14. Reed RL, Ciavarella D, Heimbach DM, et al. Prophylactic platelet administration during massive transfusion. Ann Surg 1986;203:40-8.

15. Mannuci PM, Federici AB, Sirchia G. Hemostasis testing during massive blood replacement: A study of 172 cases. Vox Sang 1982;42:113-23.

16. Pierce RN, Reich LM, Mayer K. Hemolysis following platelet transfusions from ABO-incompatible donors. Transfusion 1985;25:60-2.

17. Yankee RA, Grumet FC, Rogentine GN. Platelet transfusion therapy: The selection of compatible platelet donors for refractory patients by lymphocyte HLA typing. N Engl J Med 1969;281:1208-12.

18. Kickler TS, Braine HG, Ness PM, Koester A, Bias W. A radiolabeled antiglobulin test for crossmatching platelet transfusions. Blood 1983;61:238-42.

19. O'Connell B, Lee EJ, Schiffer CA. The value of 10-minute posttransfusion platelet counts. Transfusion 1988;28:66-7.

20. Daly PA, Schiffer CA, Aisner J, Wiernik PH. Platelet transfusion therapy: One-hour posttransfusion increments are valuable in predicting the need for HLA-matched preparations. JAMA 1980;243:435-8.

21. Bishop JF, McGrath K. Wolf MM, et al. Clinical factors influencing the efficacy of pooled platelet transfusions. Blood 1988;71:383-7.

22. Schiffer CA, Slichter ST. Platelet transfusions from single donors. N Engl J Med 1982;307:245-7.

23. Parravicini A, Rebulla P, Apuzzo J, Wenz B, Sirchia G. The preparation of leukocyte-poor red cells for transfusion by a simple cost-effective technique. Transfusion 1984;24:508-9.

24. Sirchia G, Rebulla P, Parravicini A, Carnelle V, Gianotti GA, Bertolini F. Leukocyte depletion of red cell units at the bedside by transfusion through a new filter. Transfusion 1987;27:402-5.

25. Sniecinski MR, O'Donnell B, Norwicki B, Hill LR. Prevention of refractoriness and HLA-alloimmunization using filtered blood products. Blood 1988;71:1402-7.

26. Andreu J, Dewailly C, Leberre MC, et al. Prevention of HLA immunization with leukocyte-poor packed red cells

and platelet concentrates obtained by filtration. Blood 1988;72:964-9.

27. Murphy MF, Metclafe P, Thomas H, et al. Use of leucocyte-poor blood components and HLA-matched platelet donors to prevent HLA alloimmunization. Br Med J 1986;62:529-34.

28. Dutcher JP, Schiffer CA, Aisner J, Wiernick PH. Long-term follow-up of patients with leukemia receiving platelet transfusions: Identification of a large group of patients who do not become alloimmunized. Blood 1981;58:1007-11.

29. Dausset J, Rapaport FT. Transplantation antigen activity of human blood platelets. Transplatation 1966;4:182-93.

30. Claas FHJ, Smeenk RJT, Schmidt R, van Steenbrugge GJ, Eernisse JG. Alloimmunization against the MHC antigens after platelet transfusions is due to contaminating leukocytes in the platelet suspension. Exp Hematol 1981;9:84-9.

31. Wenz B. Microaggregate blood filtration and the febrile transfusion reaction: A comparative study. Transfusion 1983;23:95-8.

32. Menitove JE, McElligott MC, Aster RH. Febrile transfusion reaction: What blood component should be given next. Vox Sang 1982;42:318-21.

33. Ernisse JG, Brand A. Prevention of platelet refractoriness due to HLA antibodies by administration of leukocyte-poor blood components. Exp Hematol 1981;9:77-83.

34. Herzig RH, Herzig GP, Bull MI, et al. Correction of pooled platelet transfusion responses with leukocyte poor HL-A matched platelet concentrates. Blood 1975;743-50.

35. Schiffer CA, Dutcher JP, Aisner J, Hogge D, Wiernik PH, Rielly JP. A randomized trial of leukocyte-depleted platelet transfusion to modify alloimmunization in patients with leukemia. Blood 1983;62:815-20.

36. Schiffer CA, Patten E, Reilly J, Patel S. Effective leukocyte removal from platelet preparations by centrifugation in new polling bag. Transfusion 1987;27:179-184.

37. Glasser L, Lane TA, McCullough J, Price TH. Neu-

trophil concentrates: Functional considerations, storage and quality control. J Clin Apheresis 1983;1:179-184.

38. Christensen RD, Rothstein G, Anstall HB, Bybee B. Granulocyte transfusions in neonates with bacterial infection, neutropenia, and depletion of mature marrow neutrophils. Pediatrics 1982;70:1-6.

39. Curnutte JT. Chronic granulomatous disease: Clinical and genetic aspects. Ann Intern Med 1988;109:134-7.

40. Winston DJ, Ho WG, Gale RP. Prophylactic granulocyte transfusions during chemotherapy of acute non-lymphocytic leukemia. Ann Int Med 1981;94:616-22.

41. Dutcher JP. Granulocyte transfusion therapy. Am J Med Sci 1984;287:11-17.

42. Strauss RG, Connett JE, Gale RP, et al. A controlled trial of prophylactic granulocyte transfusions during initial induction chemotherapy for acute myelogenous leukemia. N Engl J Med 1981;305:597-603.

43. Wolber RA, Duque RE, Robinson JP, Oberman HA. Oxidative product formation in irradiated neutrophils: A flow cytometric analysis. Transfusion 1987;27:167-70.

44. Wright DG, Robichaud KJ, Pizzo BS, Deisseroth AB. Lethal pulmonary reactions associated with the combined use of Amphotericin B and leukocyte transfusions. N Engl J Med 1981;304:1185-9.

45. Office of Medical Applications of Research. National Institutes of Health. Fresh frozen plasma: Indications and risks. JAMA 1985;253;551-3.

46. Braunstein AH, Oberman HA. Transfusion of plasma components. Transfusion 1984;24:281-6.

47. Hashim SW, Kay HR, Hammond GL, Kopf GS, Geha AS. Noncardiogenic pulmonary edema after cardiopulmonary bypass. Am J Surg 1984;147:560-4.

48. Ness PM, Perkins HA. Cryoprecipitate as a reliable source of fibrinogen replacement. JAMA 1979;241:1690-1.

49. Kitchens CS, Newcomb TF. Factor XIII. Medicine 1979;58:413-29.

50. Janson PA, Jubelirer SJ, Weinstein MJ, Deykin D. Treatment of the bleeding tendency in uremia with cryoprecipitate. N Engl J Med 1980;303:1318-22.

51. Remuzzi G. Bleeding in renal failure. Lancet 1988;1:1205-8.

52. Lupinetti FM, Stoney WS, Alford WC, et al. Cryoprecipitate: Topical thrombin glue. J. Thorac Cardiovasc Surg 1985;90:502.

53. Fischer CP, Sonda LP, Diokno AC. Use of cryoprecipitate coagulum in extracting renal calculi. Urology 1980;15:6-13.

54. Human Factor VIII:C purified using monoclonal antibody to von Willebrand factor. Semin Hematol 1988;25:(2):Suppl.1.

55. Brettler DB, Forsberg AD, Levine PH, Petillo J, Lamon K, and Sullivan JL. Factor VIII:C concentrate purified from plasma using monoclonal antibodies: Human Studies. Blood 1989;73:1859-63.

56. White GC II, McMillan CW, Kingdom HS, Shoemaker CB. Use of recombinant antihemophilic factor in the treatment of two patients with classic hemophilia. N Engl J Med 1989;320:166-70.

57. International Forum. Ways to reduce the risk of transmission of viral infections by plasma and plasma products: A comparison of methods, their advantages and disadvantages. Vox Sang 1988;54:228-45.

58. Brettler DB, Levine PH. Factor concentrates for treatment of hemophilia: Which one to choose? Blood 1989;73:2067-73.

59. Zauber NP, Levin J. Factor IX levels in patients with hemophilia B (Christmas disease) following transfusion with concentrates of factor IX or fresh frozen plasma (FFP). Medicine 1977;56:213-24.

60. Lusher JM. Management of patients with factor VIII inhibitors, Transf Med Rev 1987;1:123-30.

61. Hilgartner MW, Knatterud GL, FEIBA Study Group. The use of factor eight inhibitor bypassing activity (FEIBA IMMUNO) product for treatment of bleeding episodes in hemophiliacs with inhibitors. Blood 1982;61:36-40.

62. Tullis JL. Albumin 2. Guidelines for clinical use. JAMA 1977;237:460-3.

63. Snyder E. Clinical use of albumin, plasma protein fraction and isoimmune globulin products. In: Silvergleid A, Britten A, eds. Plasma products: Use and management. Arlington, VA: American Association of Blood Banks, 1982:87-107.

64. Olinger GN, Werner PH, Boncheck LI, et al. Vasodilator effects of the sodium acetate in pooled protein fraction. Ann Surg 1979;190:305-11.

65. Cervera AL, Moss G. Crystalloid distribution following hemorrhage and hemodilution; mathematical model and prediction of optimum volumes for equilibration at normovolemia. J Trauma 1974;14:506-20.

66. Moss GS, Gould S. Plasma expanders—an update. Surg Pharmacol 1988;155:425-34.

67. Berkman SA, Lee ML, Gale RP. Clinical uses intravenous immunoglobulins. Semin Hematol 1988;25:140-58.

68. Romer J, Morgenthaler JJ, Scherz, et al. Characterization of various immunoglobulin preparations for intravenous application 1. Protein composition and antibody content. Vox Sang 1982;42:62-73.

69. Boshkov LK, Kelton JG. Use of intravenous gamma globulin as an immune replacement and an immune suppressant. Transf Med Rev 1989;3:82-120.

70. Buckley RH. Immunoglobulin replacement therapy: Indications and contraindications for use and variable IgG levels achieved. In: Alving BM, Finlayson JS, eds. Immunoglobulins: Characteristics and use of intravenous preparations. Washington, DC: US Department of Health and Human Services, 1979:3-8.

71. Warrier I, Lusher JM. Intravenous gamma globulin treatment for chronic idiopathic thrombocytopenic purpura in children. Am J Med 1984;76(3a):193-8.

72. Nydegger UE. New aspects of immunoglobulin treatment for idiopathic thrombocytopenic purpura. Plas Ther Transf Technol 1988;9:83-7.

73. Bossell J, et al. Safety of therapeutic immune globulin preparations with respect to transmission of human T lymphotropic virus type III/LAV infection. MMWR 1986;35:231-3.

74. Bussel J, Cunningham-Rundles C, Feldman C, Horowitz B. Transmission of viral infection by preparation of intravenous immunoglobulin. Plas Ther Transf Technol 1988;9:193-205.

75. Weiland O, Mattsson L, Glaumann H. Non-A, non-B hepatitis after intravenous gamma globulin. Lancet 1986;1:976-7.

76. American College of Obstetrics and Gynecology. Prevention of Rho(D) isoimmunization. ACOG Tech Bulletin 1984;79:1-4.

77. Proceedings of the McMaster Conference on prevention of Rh immunization. Vox Sang 1979;36:50-64.

78. Bowman JM. Suppression of Rh isoimmunization—a review. Obstet Gynecol 1978;52:385-93.

79. Lack of transmission of human immunodeficiency virus through Rho(D) immune globulin (human). MMWR 1987;36(44).

80. Salama A, Kiefel V, Amberg R, et al. Treatment of autoimmune thrombocytopenia purpura with rhesus antibodies [anti-Rho(D)]. Blut 1984;49:29-35.

81. Pollack W, Gorman JG, Freda VJ. Rh immune suppression: Past, present and future. In: Frigoletto FJ, Jewett JF, Konygres AA, eds. Rh hemolytic disease. New strategy for eradication. Boston: GK Hall, 1982:58-9.

82. Hultin MA, McKay J, Abildgaard U. Antithrombin Oslo: Type 1b classification of the first reported-deficient family, with a review of hereditary antithrombin variants. Thromb Haemost 1988;59:468-73.

83. Wewers MD, Casolaro MA, Sellers SE, et al. Replacement therapy for alpha$_1$-antitrypsin deficiency associated with emphysema. N Engl J Med 1987;316:1055-62.

84. Garver RI Jr, Mornex J-F, Nukiwa T, et al. Alpha$_1$-antitrypsin deficiency and emphysema caused by homozygous inheritance of non-expressing alpha$_1$-antitrypsin genes. N Engl J Med 1986;314:762-6.

85. Cohen AB. Unraveling the mysteries of alpha$_1$-antitrypsin deficiency. N Engl J Med 1986;314:778-9.

86. Gould SA, Rosen AL, Sehgal LR. Fluosol-DA as a red cell substitute in acute anemia. N Engl J Med 1986;314:1653-6.

87. Zanjani ED, Ascenao JL. Erythropoietin. Transfusion 1989;29:46-57.

88. Winearls CG, Oliver DO, Pippard MJ, Reid C, Downing MR, Cotes PM. Effect of human erythropoietin derived from recombinant DNA on the anaemia of patients maintained by chronic haemodialysis. Lancet 1986;2:1175-8.

89. Eschbach JW, Egric JC, Downing MR, Browne JK,

Adamson JW. Correction of the anemia of end stage renal disease with recombinant human erythropoietin. Results of a combined phase I and II clinical trial. N Engl J Med 1987;316:73-8.

90. Clinical applications of hematopoietic growth factors. Semin Hematol 1989;26:(2):Suppl.2.

91. Friedman BA. An analysis of surgical blood use in United States hospitals with applications to the maximum surgical blood order schedule. Transfusion 1979;19:268-78.

92. Mintz PD, Nordine RB, Henry JB, Webb WR. Expected hemotherapy in elective surgery. NYS J Med 1976; 76:532-7.

93. Oberman HA, Barnes BA, Friedman BA. The risk of abbreviating the major crossmatch in urgent or massive transfusion. Transfusion 1978;18:137-41.

94. Silvergleid AJ. Safety and effectiveness of predeposit autologous transfusions in preteen and adolescent children. JAMA 1987;257:3403-4.

95. Wentworth L, Pura L, Pepkowitz S, et al. Obstetrical autologous donors. Transfusion 1987;27:573.

96. Grossman BJ, Stewart NC, Grindon AJ. Increased risk of positive test for anti-HBc in autologous donors. Transfusion 1987;27:523.

97. Collins JA. Massive blood transfusions. Clin Haematol 1976;5:201-22.

98. Mannucci PM, Federici AB, Sirchia G. Hemostasis testing during massive blood replacement. Vox Sang 1982;42:113-23.

99. Shackford SR, Virgilio R, Peters RM. Whole blood versus packed-cell transfusions. Ann Surg 1981;193: 337-40.

100. Ciavarella D, Reed RL, Counts RB, et al. Clotting factor levels and the risk of diffuse microvascular bleeding in the massively transfused patient. Br J Haematol 1987;67:365-8.

101. Grannum PA, Copel JA, Plaxe SC, et al. In utero exchange transfusion by direct intravascular injection in severe erythroblastosis fetalis. N Engl J Med 1986;314:1431-4.

102. Kim HC. Red cell transfusion in the neonate. Semin. Perinatol 1983;2:114-8.
103. Ludvigsen C, Swanson J, Thompson T, McCullough J. Failure of neonates to form red cell antibodies following transfusion (abstract). Transfusion 1982;22:405.
104. Yeager A, Grumet F, Hafleight E, Arvin A, et al. Prevention of transfusion acquired cytomegalovirus infections in newborn infants. J Pediatr 1981;98:281-7.
105. Adler S, Chandrika T, Lawrence L, Baggett J. Cytomegalovirus infections in neonates acquired by blood transfusion. Ped Infect Dis 1983;2:114-8.
106. Leitman SF, Holland PV. Irradiation of blood products: indications and guidelines. Transfusion 1985;25: 293-300.
107. Welch HG, Larson EB, Slichter SJ. Providing platelets for refractory patients: Prudent strategies. Transfusion 1989;29:193-5.
108. Bolgiano DC, Larson EB, Slichter SJ. A model to determine required pool size for HLA-typed community donor apheresis programs. Transfusion 1989;29:306-10.
109. Duquesnoy RJ, Filip DJ, Rodney GE, Rimm AA, Aster RH. Successful transfusion of platelets ''mismatched'' for HLA antigens to alloimmunized thrombocytopenic patients. Am J Hematol 1977;2:219-26.
110. Dahlke MB, Weiss KL. Platelet transfusion from donors mismatched for crossreactive HLA antigens. Transfusion 1984;24:299-302.
111. Murphy S. ABO groups and platelet transfusion. Transfusion 1988;28:401-2.
112. Freedman J, Garvey MB, Salomon de Friedberg Z, Hornstein A, Blanchette V. Random donor platelet crossmatching: Comparison of four platelet antibody detection methods. Am J Hematol 1988;28:1-7.
113. Aster RH. New approaches to an old problem: Refractoriness to platelet transfusions. Transfusion 1988; 28:95-6.
114. Storb R, Thomas ED, Buckner CD, et al. Marrow transplantation in thirty ''untransfused'' patients with severe aplastic anemia. Ann Intern Med 1980;92:30-6.
115. Leivestad T. Flatmark A, Thorsby E. Influence of donor-specific transfusion in recipients of one HLA hap-

lotype matched related donor. Kidney Transplant Proc 1985;17:2357-61.

116. Cats S, Terasaki P, Perdue S, et al. Effect of HLA typing and transfusions on cyclosporine-treated renal-allograft recipients. N Engl J Med 1984;311:675-6.

117. Buchholz DH, Lin A, Snyder E, et al. Plasma separation using a hollow fiber membrane device. Transfusion 1986;26:145-50.

118. Applications Committee, American Society for Apheresis. Clinical applications of therapeutic apheresis. J Clin Apheresis 1986;3:93-9.

119. Edelson R. Berger C, Gasparro F, et al. Treatment of cutaneous T-cell lymphoma by extracorporeal photochemotherapy. Preliminary results. N Engl J Med 1987;316:297-303.

120. Klein HJ, ed. Clinical application of therapeutic apheresis—report of the clinical applications committee of the American Society for Apheresis. J Clin Apheresis 1986;3:1-92.

121. AMA Panel on Therapeutic Plasmapheresis. Current status of therapeutic plasmapheresis and related techniques. JAMA 1985;253:819-25.

122. International Forum. What are the established clinical indications for therapeutic plasma exchange and how important is the choice of replacement fluid for efficacy of therapeutic plasma exchange in these situations? Vox Sang 1982;43:270-95.

123. Boyan CP, Howland WS. Cardiac arrest and temperature of bank blood. JAMA 1963;183:58-60.

124. Arens JF, Leonard GL. Danger of overwarming blood by microwave. JAMA 1971;218:1045-6.

125. Ryden SE, Oberman HA. Compatibility of common intravenous solutions with CPD blood. Transfusion 1975;15:250-5.

126. Snyder EL, Bookbinder M. Role of microaggregate blood filtration in clinical medicine. Transfusion 1983;23:460-70.

127. Snyder EL, Hezzey A, Barash G, Palermo G. Microaggregate blood filtration in patients with compromised pulmonary function. Transfusion 1982;22:21-5.

128. Snyder EL, Ferri PM, Smith EO, Ezekowitz MD. Use of

an electromechanical infusion pump for transfusion of platelet concentrates. Transfusion 1984;24:524-7.

129. Snyder EL, Malech HL, Ferri PM, Gardner JP, Kalish R. In vitro function of granulocyte concentrates following passage through an electromechanical infusion pump. Transfusion 1986;26:141-4.

130. Tomasulo PA. Platelet transfusion for nonmalignant diseases. In: Petz LD, Swisher SN, eds. 1st ed. Clinical practice of blood transfusion. New York: Churchill Livingstone, 1981:529.

131. Fernandez F, Goudable C, Sie P, et al. Low hematocrit and prolonged bleeding time in uremic patients: Effect of red cell transfusions. Br J Haemaol 1985;59:139-48.

132. Harker LA, Malpass TW, Branson HE, et al. Mechanism of abnormal bleeding in patients undergoing cardiopulmonary bypass: Acquired transient platelet dysfunction associated with selective alpha granule release. Blood 1980;56:824-34.

133. Eisenberg JM, Clarke JR, Sussman SA. Prothrombin and partial thromboplastin time as preoperative screening tests. Arch Surg 1982;117:48-51.

134. Kobrinsky NL, Gerrard JM, Watson CM, et al. Shortening of bleeding time by 1-deamino-8-D-arginine vasopressin in various bleeding disorders. Lancet 1984;1:1145-8.

135. Ruggeri ZM, Mannucci PM, Lombardi R, et al. Multimeric composition of factor VIII/von Willebrand factor following administration of DDAVP: Implications for pathophysiology and therapy of von Willebrand's disease subtypes. Blood 1982;59:1272-8.

136. Schipper HG, Ten Cate JW. Antithrombin III transfusion in patients with hepatic cirrhosis. Br J Haematol 1982;52:25-33.

137. Clonse LH, Comp PC. The regulation of hemostasis: the protein C system. N Engl J Med 1986;314:1298-1304.

138. American College of Physicians. Thrombolysis for evolving myocardial infarction. Ann Intern Med 1985;103:463-9.

139. Jaffe AS, Sobel BE. Thrombolysis with tissue-type plasminogen activator in acute myocardial infarction. JAMA 1986;255:237-9.

140. Pineda AA, Brzica SM, Taswell HF. Hemolytic transfusion reaction—recent experience in a large blood bank. Mayo Clin Proc 1978;53:378-90.

141. Yap PL, Pryde EAD, McCelland DBL. IgA content of frozen-thawed-washed red blood cells and blood products measured by radioimmunoassay. Transfusion 1982;22:36-8.

142. Ward HN. Pulmonary infiltrates associated with leukoagglutinin transfusion reactions. Ann Intern Med 1970;73:689-94.

143. Dubois M, Lotze MT, Diamond WJ, Kim YD, Flye MW, MacNamara TE. Pulmonary shunting during leukoagglutinin-induced noncardiac pulmonary edema. JAMA 1980;244:2186-9.

144. Popovsky MA, Abel MD, Moore SG. Transfusion related acute lung injury associated with passive transfer of antileukocyte antibodies. Am Rev Resp Dis 1983; 128:185-9.

145. Tabor E, Gerety RJ. Five cases of pseudomonas sepsis transmitted by blood transfusion. Lancet 1984;1:1403.

146. Wright DC, Selss IF, Vinton KJ, Pierce RN. Fatal Yersinia enterocolitica sepsis after blood transfusion. Arch Pathol Lab Med 1985;109:1040-2.

147. Khabbaz RF, Arnow PM, Highsmith AK, Herwaldt LA, Chou T, Jarvis WR, Lerche NW, Allen JR. Pseudomonas fluorescens bacteremia from blood transfusion. Am J Med 1984;76:62-8.

148. Heal JM, Jones ME, Forey J, et al. Fatal *Salmonella* septicemia after platelet transfusion. Transfusion 1987; 27:2-5.

149. Arnow PM, Weiss LM, Weil D, Rosen NR. Escherichia coli sepsis from contaminated platelet transfusion. Arch Intern Med 1986;146:321-4.

150. Goldbert LI. Cardiovascular and renal actions of dopamine: potential clinical applications. Pharm Rev 1972;24:1-29.

151. Lostumbo MM, Holland PV, Schmidt PJ. Isoimmunization after multiple transfusions. N Engl J Med 1966;275:141-4.

152. Aach RD, Kahn RA. Posttransfusion hepatitis—current perspectives. Ann Intern Med 1980;92:539-46.

153. Seeff LB, Wright EC, Zimmerman HJ, McCollum RW, and Members of VA Hepatitis Cooperative Studies Group. VA cooperative study of post-transfusion hepatitis, 1969-1974: incidence and characteristics of hepatitis and responsible risk factors. Am J Med Sci 1975;270:355-62.

154. National Institutes of Health Consensus development conference: Perioperative red blood cell transfusion. JAMA 1988;260:2700-3.

155. Curran JW, Lawrence DN, Jaffe H, et al. Acquired immunodeficiency syndrome (AIDS) associated with transfusion. N Engl J Med 1984;310:69-75.

156. Melief CJM, Goudsmit J. Transmission of lymphotropic retroviruses (HTLV-I and LAV/HTLV-III) by blood transfusion and blood products. Vox Sang 1986;50:1-11.

157. Lang DJ, Ebert PA, Rodgers M. Boggess HP, Rixse RS. Reduction of postperfusion cytomegalovirus infection following the use of leukocyte depleted blood. Transfusion 1977;17:391-5.

158. Guerrerro IC, Weniger BC, Schultz MG. Transfusion malaria in the United States, 1972-1981. Ann Intern Med 1983;99:221-6.

159. Siegel SE, Lunde MN, Gelderman AH, et al. Transmission of toxoplasmosis by leukocyte transfusion. Blood 1971;37:388-94.

160. Jacobs A. Iron chelation therapy for iron loaded patients. Br J Haematol 1979;43:1-5.

161. Von Fliedner V, Higby DJ, Kim V. Graft-versus-host reaction following blood product transfusion. Am J Med 1982;72:951-61.

Recommended Readings

Biggs R, Rizza CR. Human blood coagulation, haemostasis and thrombosis, 3rd ed. Oxford: Blackwell Scientific Publications, 1984.

Walker RH, ed. Technical manual, 10th ed. Arlington, VA: American Association of Blood Banks, 1989 (in press).

American Medical Association. General principles of blood transfusion, revised edition. Chicago:AMA, 1985.

Mollison PL. Blood transfusion in clinical medicine, 8th ed. Oxford: Blackwell Scientific Publications, 1987.

Coleman RW, Hirsh J, Marder VJ, Salzman EW. Hemostasis and thrombosis, basic principles and clinical practice, 2nd ed. Philadelphia: JB Lippincott, 1987.

Huestis DW, Bove JR, Case J. Practical blood transfusion, 4th ed. Boston: Little, Brown and Company, 1987.

Petz LD, Swisher SN. Clinical practice of transfusion medicine, 2nd ed. New York: Churchill Livingston, 1989.

Journals

American Journal of Hematology

Blood

British Journal of Haematology

Clinics in Hematology

Journal of Clinical Apheresis

Progress in Transfusion Medicine

Seminars in Hematology

Seminars in Thrombosis and Hemostasis

Transfusion

Transfusion Medicine Reviews

Vox Sanguinis

Index

(Page numbers in italics indicate tables.)

Ringer's lactate, 36

S

Salvaged blood, 48-50
Scheduling, MSBOS, 47
Shelf life, 1, 49, 50
Storage, whole blood, 5, *5*
    See also Red cells, frozen-
        thawed-deglycerolized
Streptokinase, 75

T

Temperature, blood warming,
   64
Tissue-type plasminogen
   activator (t-PA), 76
Transfusion reactions, acute,
   77, *82-83*
    investigation, 80
    treatment, 80

Transfusion reactions, delayed,
   82, 84-85
Transfusion, time limits for, 65
Transplantation, 60
Type and screen, 47

U-Z

Urticaria, 78, 81
Urokinase, 75
Vitamin K deficiency, 73
Volume expanders, synthetic
    administration, 37
    composition, 36
    indications, 36
    side effects and
        precautions, 37
von Willebrand's disease, 28,
   71
Warfarin-induced
   coagulopathy, 73
Zoster immune globulin, 39